THE
MASTER
CLEANSE
EXPERIENCE

D1016503

THE
MASTER
CLEANSE
EXPERIENCE

Day-to-Day Accounts
of What to Expect
and How to Succeed
on The Lemonade Diet

Introduction by
TOM WOLOSHYN

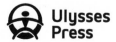

Ulysses
Press

Published by: Ulysses Press
P.O. Box 3440
Berkeley, CA 94703
www.ulyssespress.com

ISBN: 978-1-56975-708-6
Library of Congress Control Number: 2008911759

Printed in the United States by Bang Printing

10 9 8 7 6 5 4 3 2 1

Acquisitions Editor: Nicholas Denton-Brown
Managing Editor: Claire Chun
Editor: Keith Riegert
Copyeditors: Hope Richardson, Lily Chou
Proofreader: Lily Chou
Production: Judith Metzener
Front cover design: what!design @ whatweb.com
Cover photo: ©istockphoto.com
Journal contributors: Ella Benson, Samantha A. Cooper, Queen Jahneen Etter, Christy Hall, Joann Kim, Nalea Ko, Flash Mallach, Genevieve Melzer, Noel N., Kimberly Padgett, Susan Williams, Holly Wisniewski

Distributed by Publishers Group West

"MASTER CLEANSE" is used in the title and contents of this book in its generic sense as a term for a detoxification diet that has been widely used and discussed since it was first introduced in 1941. This book is an independent work of information and commentary and is not affiliated with, or sponsored or endorsed by, any manufacturer of consumables or other goods and services.

NOTE TO READERS
This book has been written and published strictly for informational and educational purposes only. It is not intended to serve as medical advice or to be any form of medical treatment. You should always consult your physician before altering or changing any aspect of your medical treatment and/or undertaking a diet regimen, including the Master Cleanse diet as described in this book. Do not stop or change any prescription medications without the guidance and advice of your physician. Any use of the information in this book is made on the reader's good judgment after consulting with his or her physician and is the reader's sole responsibility. This book is not intended to diagnose or treat any medical condition and is not a substitute for a physician.

Contents

Why Keep a Master Cleanse Journal?

Life on the Master Cleanse

In deciding to read this book, you've taken the first big step on the road to a life-altering Master Cleanse experience. You're probably aware that the Master Cleanse is a rigorous mono diet consisting of fresh-squeezed lemons, cayenne pepper and maple syrup—likely the polar opposite of the diet you follow now. Given that fact, the week and a half looming ahead is bound to be a difficult and challenging experience. Ten days on a liquid diet is no hundred-yard dash—it's the dietary version of a marathon.

One of the most intense trials you're likely to endure in your first few days of the Master Cleanse is that while you embark on the body- and soul-revolutionizing cleanse, life goes on as normal all around you. Indeed, Master Cleansers say the hardest part about the cleanse is that you invariably go it alone. At work, you'll be surrounded by people sipping coffee, snacking on pastries, eating lunch. Then you'll come home only to be tempted again by the aroma of your spouse or roommates cooking dinner. All the while, you'll be gulping down lemonade by the quart, along with laxative tea and the occasional saltwater flush. This is no picnic. The lack of energy, flushing of your digestive tract and monotony of consumption can cause frustration that needs an avenue for release. Turn to the journal! With such a great outlet for self-expression, plus a little support, determination and careful organization, those ten days will fly by.

Using This Book

Whether you're attempting your first cleanse or your fourteenth, journaling may make the difference between a successful cleanse and a Day Four binge on french fries. The majority of "cleansers" embark on those tough ten days alone. Even those who are fortunate enough to find a cleansing companion say the process is daunting. With such a radical transformation in diet it's hard to get a clear idea of what's happening to your body, what your expectations should be and whether or not the things you're experiencing are normal. Having some sense of what the cleanse is like for others is extraordinarily helpful. To try to clear up that picture, we've collected journals from across the country that represent a range of different experiences and perspectives. We hope this will help demystify the Master Cleanse, and perhaps even provide a little camaraderie to make the challenge less isolating.

As you make your way through your cleanse day by day, follow along with the journals. You may find these cleansers went through the same experiences you're facing right now.

Keeping Your Own Journal

You should treat your Master Cleanse journal as a mixture of an intimate personal diary and a fascinating scientific record. Chances are, this is one of the most intense transformations you'll ever put your body through. Keeping a record of the experience not only documents a great personal triumph, but it can make the difference between success and failure by giving you strict organization and a fantastic way to vent! Here's how to get started.

Record everything. That's the advice most cleansers give when it comes to keeping a journal. Along with the triumphs—how many pounds you've shed and how much energy you have gained—take serious notes about the tribulations, including those unmentionable bodily functions. You don't want to forget this radical transformation.

Keep track of your goals. If you set out to lose ten pounds on your Master Cleanse diet, make sure you're weighing yourself daily and recording your progress. Keep in mind, weight loss can be frustrating on the liquid intensive cleanse as your body's water weight will shift daily. Don't let raw numbers get you down; make sure you're recording how you *feel,* not just what the scale reads.

Write down the tools you need for confidence. A huge part of getting through the Master Cleanse is summoning the mental strength and confidence to do it. *The Complete Master Cleanse* details how important it is to create affirmations to assist your body in letting go of the waste it has accumulated. The mind-body connection runs extraordinarily deep and just writing and repeating your positive thought patterns can make all the difference during difficult moments.

Keep an eye on your emotions. The rigors of the cleanse can be emotionally trying. On top of that, your body's physical chemistry changes as you release toxins, often leading to some hormonal turbulence. You may just find that your cleanse is affecting those around you almost as much as it affects you. Treat your journal like your own personal confidant; record your ups, downs and rocky in-betweens. Chances are your friends and family will be grateful.

Take note of your energy levels. Probably the most radically noticeable change during the cleanse is your daily stamina. Many cleansers report plummeting energy levels during the first few days of the cleanse, followed by remarkably high levels toward the end, as the body adjusts to the strict diet.

Follow up with a couple of days after the cleanse. Your Master Cleanse experience probably won't end with your final glass of lemonade. Reintroducing food to your body is not only a bit of a challenge, it's a fantastic opportunity to pay attention to what your body wants and needs. Pay careful attention to what foods you can digest easily and what foods your body would rather not have. The more you listen, the more your diet will improve in the future. And remember, write everything down; chances are two weeks after your cleanse is over, you won't recall how those first few meals felt.

PART 1
Introduction: The Master Cleanse in Review

If you have not yet done your Master Cleanse, this section will serve as a primer to help guide you through the ten days of diet transformation. However, these are just the very basic elements of the Master Cleanse. For more in-depth information, you should follow the detailed instructions in *The Complete Master Cleanse* or *Beyond the Master Cleanse*.

Benefits of the Cleanse

Over my many years of practice, people have reported myriad benefits that occur during or after a Master Cleanse. To give only the principal ones:

Better sleep—Sleep becomes deeper and more restful.

More energy—Those who complete the cleanse experience report increased energy to the point where some people start following an exercise program, even though they have never exercised in their lives.

Clarity of mind—People tell me that a burst of awareness has come over them, almost frightening them, because after a cleanse they realize how out of touch they were with their bodies and their overall health.

Positive outlook—One woman called to thank me for my help with her cleanse because she no longer harbored thoughts of suicide.

Greater flexibility—Even yoga instructors who have done a cleanse have told me how astonished they were at their increased physical flexibility.

Weight loss—Women often lose one pound per day during a cleanse, men up to two pounds.

Freedom from addictions—I have known many people who stop smoking, using alcohol, doing recreational drugs or consuming junk foods.

Increased strength—During and after a cleanse, many people who like to work out are able to increase their weight load when at the gym.

Reduced pain and swelling—These conditions are often alleviated.

Healthier scalp and hair—People report their hair stops falling out and increases in body.

Better skin—Problem skin clears up and becomes healthier.

Allergy relief—Some allergies are significantly lessened, and others even disappear entirely after a cleanse or two.

You may experience many more positive outcomes from doing the Master Cleanse!

First, mentally prepare yourself for the cleanse and all that it involves. Be aware that whenever people start a Master Cleanse on a whim, they tend to go off it on a whim. It lacks importance to them, so it's no wonder they fail on it. Therefore, it's best to set a goal of at least ten days on the Master Cleanse. Set those days aside and make sure you don't have a full calendar of social events. It usually is best not to tell too many people (or sometimes anyone outside your own home) that you are doing a cleanse.

Second, do not let others discourage you. I have seen many prospective cleanses aborted because of the misguided advice of third-party doubters. These skeptics have never done the Master Cleanse or, if they have done it, did it incorrectly. Do not let others sabotage your efforts. You'll want to surround yourself with people who support you in your journey toward greater wellness.

How to Get Started

Some people like to prepare their body before a cleanse. They go on a primarily vegetarian diet for four or five days, then ramp up to an all-veggie diet before starting the cleanse itself. This simpler diet will be less stressful on the body and will make it easier for you to transition to the Master Cleanse. It may also help you on the path to making better food choices in the long run.

If you drink coffee or caffeinated soda every day, you will want to prevent the headaches that are caused by caffeine withdrawal. Start taking pantothenic acid (vitamin B-5) about four days before starting the cleanse. The dosage should be approximately 400 mg, taken three times a day, while at the same time you reduce your coffee or soda intake about 25 percent each day. This will help you taper off the caffeine that you are accustomed to having. The day you start your cleanse, you will be off coffee or soda completely and will no longer need to take the vitamin supplement.

Most importantly, you will need to go out and gather your ingredients: lemons, maple syrup, cayenne pepper, herbal laxatives and sea salt. (See the sections below for full details and properties of all ingredients.) If you have no other source of good water, you will need to add bottled water to your list. Whenever possible, buy organic lemons to make your lemonade drink; it will taste much better and will also have a higher nutritional quality since it won't have been treated by pesticides, herbicides or chemical fertilizers that are typically used in commercially grown produce. Some consumers might complain about the higher cost of organic produce, but remember that this is the only food you will be eating for ten days or more—so get the best; you deserve it.

Contraindications and Cautions

People who have had organ transplants and are on immune-suppressant drugs *cannot* do the Master Cleanse. The cleanse will stimulate the immune system and also inhibit the effectiveness of the drugs, a combination that will likely cause the immune system to attack the transplanted organ and end in serious—and possibly dangerous—problems.

Issues with Lemons or Cayenne

The Master Cleanse uses lemons and cayenne, precisely because they possess properties that are good for stirring up toxicity in the body. Their effects, however, are often mislabeled or misunderstood. If you are already somewhat toxic and you are eating either lemons or cayenne or both and experiencing discomfort or what you think is an allergic reaction, this may be due to your body's simultaneous attempt to cleanse itself *and* digest food. This creates a conflict; sometimes it even causes severe discomfort. When you are on the Master Cleanse you are not eating any other foods, so the issue of other food allergies does not arise.

Surrender to the Process

It can be hard to try something entirely new, especially if it's something that sounds a bit weird or perhaps risky—even though you hear good things about it from people you trust. You might try this little mental exercise that I often give to clients who are anxious. On first glance it seems odd, but it works:

1. *Know where you are.* Imagine that you have called a travel agent and are asking her to book you a flight, but you have no idea where you are! This is a disconcerting feeling, so avoid it by taking the time to center yourself.

2. *Know where you are going.* Again call the travel agent and say, "I am in Seattle but I don't want to go to New York or Miami, not to Atlanta, either. I also don't like London as a destination." The agent, in frustration, will ask, "Well, where *do* you want to go?"

3. *Surrender to the process.* You know where you are and where you want to go. You now have to trust the travel agent, the airline, the taxi driver, the baggage handler and all concerned that they will get you and your suitcase to your destination. The agent will ask for the dates you want to travel and for payment. Your only responsibility is to show up at the airport at the right time on the proper day, and as if by magic you will soon arrive at your destination. You do not have to design the plane, build, fuel or fly it. *You just get on the plane!* You surrender to the process that others have established and tested.

Now apply this exercise to your current state of health and the goals you desire to achieve by using the Master Cleanse. Start by surveying your present state of health. Once you know where you are, move on to the next step—defining the results you want.

As you think about your first Master Cleanse, be flexible and open-minded about it, just as you would if you were flying overseas for the first time and feeling a little anxious. In both situations you could meet a little turbulence or have to change flights partway there, or be bothered a bit by rough weather. Just trust yourself and be willing to roll with whatever comes up.

Don't get upset or disturbed if every little thing doesn't happen exactly the way you might expect. This process can be exciting and adventurous. This journey toward better health may change your life—it will almost surely bring you much more than you imagine.

It just so happens that I am writing this paragraph on the exact day when, twenty-seven years ago, I was taking a course on Stanley Burroughs's work. Did I know that first step would start me on the long road to where I am today? No, but I did know it was absolutely the thing I wanted to do—so I surrendered myself to doing it with a happy heart.

How to Do the Master Cleanse

Again, while this section of the book is a helpful tool for doing the Master Cleanse, it is geared more toward giving you an idea of what the Master Cleanse entails to help guide you through your cleanse with greater ease. You should read *The Complete Master Cleanse* from cover to cover to ensure absolute success on your first Master Cleanse. Make notes or highlight steps, cautions and tips you feel are especially helpful.

Make sure you understand how to do the Master Cleanse properly so that you can complete it with success and experience the benefits. I'm amused to recall that Stanley Burroughs would often say something that technical support people still tell their frustrated customers: "WAEFFTI—When All Else Fails, Follow The Instructions."

GOOD TO READ

Some readers might profit from browsing through Stanley Burroughs's original small volume, *Healing for the Age of Enlightenment*. The author self-published it in 1976; it was revised and reprinted in 1993. Though the book is sometimes out of print, a limited number of copies may be available through used bookstores or an online book vendor.

Follow these steps, in order (they are explained at length in the sections below).

1. Gather the ingredients.

2. Take an herbal laxative the night before you start the cleanse.

3. The next morning, repeat the laxative or drink an internal saltwater bath.

4. Be sure to have three or four bowel movements every day while using the laxative.

5. Now start to drink the lemonade, freshly made: six to twelve glasses each day.

Step 1 — Gather Ingredients

First, assemble all the ingredients you need to do your cleanse. Buy only enough lemons for about three days at a time if you can. (You will need a total of approximately sixty to one hundred lemons, depending on their size, for a ten-day cleanse.) If you wish to use limes instead of lemons, make sure that they are ripe and starting to be yellow in color; a dark green lime is unripe.

A close friend did the Master Cleanse using only green, unripe limes and after several days complained that she felt sick with every glass of limeade she drank. Limes that have developed brown spots become bitter tasting and should not be used.

It is best to keep lemons on a counter at room temperature, or to even set them in the sunlight; this allows them to ripen. I check my lemons and limes once or twice a day to make sure they are not

> **Shopping List**
>
> To prepare ingredients for the full cleanse, you will need the following (approximately):
> - 60 to 80 (organic) lemons
> - 2 quarts maple syrup
> - ½ cup sea salt
> - 10 gallons of good water (more if you want to drink it both as water and as tea)
> - 2 ounces cayenne pepper
> - Sufficient herbal laxative
> - Set of measuring spoons

starting to spoil. If they are ripening too quickly, I rub a small amount of lemon essential oil on the lemon or lime peel to prevent spoilage.

Lemons and limes kept in the refrigerator will have a lower enzyme activity (which you don't want) and be less flavorful. If you have refrigerated lemons, remove them about two days before you use them.

Step 2—Take an Herbal Laxative

With the ingredients all assembled, you will begin the Master Cleanse by taking an herbal laxative the night before you start. The laxative may be in the form of a tablet, capsule or tea. If you prefer tea, make it according to instructions, but make a note of how strong it turns out; it may need to be steeped longer, or to have another tea bag added, to strengthen its effects. When using the laxative in tablet or capsule form, you generally need at least three to five of them to create the desired results.

Whatever the form you take it in, the laxative must be used each and every night of the Master Cleanse. This will ensure that you eliminate all the toxins that your body is releasing.

The laxative may cause diarrhea symptoms in some people. If this occurs, stop taking it until the diarrhea has stopped. Please remember that this is a liquid mono diet, with no fiber whatsoever to bulk up in the colon. The continual ingestion of fluids, combined with the elimination of runny, slimy mucus and old waste, will make your bowel movements appear as though you have diarrhea. (In fact, you may not.) It can take two to three days for the stool to go from firm to rather loose. The diarrhea symptoms I am speaking of are manifested when you have to run repeatedly to the bathroom several times a day without much control of your colon.

Step 3 — Repeat the Laxative, or Drink a Saltwater Bath

In the morning of Day One of the cleanse, before drinking lemonade, *either* repeat taking the herbal laxative *or* use an internal saltwater bath. The internal saltwater bath is made by adding two teaspoons of *non*iodized sea salt to one quart of warm water. The saltwater is mixed to the same salinity as your blood. When you drink this mixture, the salinity keeps the water from being absorbed into the bloodstream. You will not absorb the salt unless you are deficient in salt or the many trace minerals it contains. The saltwater normally passes into the colon and out the rectum.

You can drink the saltwater bath every morning, or can omit it completely if you use the laxative instead. There are several considerations to weigh before making your choice. First, keep in mind that the saltwater bath acts quickly: it can start to be eliminated within half an hour, or can take up to one and a half hours to take effect after you drink it. The final elimination of the saltwater will often come about one hour after your first elimination.

The upside to the saltwater bath is that, after the first few hours, you will not have to make any urgent runs to the bathroom throughout the rest of the day. This is very helpful if, for example, you plan to be in a dentist's chair or in a business meeting during the day, or are traveling on an airplane (though you will try to avoid that). Occasionally, someone will not pass the saltwater on their initial attempts. If this happens, don't worry about it; just add more salt the next time.

The herbal laxative can cause cramping. This is usually the result of your colon discharging some rather nasty stuff. At a certain point you will not want to overdo the laxative because it may cause severe cramping, even nausea. However, I find that, for me, the laxative is better at eliminating waste from the colon, so I usually do the saltwater bath only three times in a ten-day cleanse. I drink the saltwater on Day One, then again on Day Three or Four, and finally on Day Seven or Eight.

I have taken the internal saltwater bath hundreds of times, and I find it pleasant to do. Please do *not* drink the quart or liter of saltwater all at one time, as you will probably throw it up and be disgusted with it. I take about ten minutes to drink my saltwater, and I warm it to body temperature before consuming it. Some people imagine they are drinking a salty soup or broth, which seems to work for them. You may find the saltwater distasteful at first, but after a short time you should get used to it and it will become easy to swallow.

Step 4—Have Daily Bowel Movements

It is vital that you have at least three to four eliminations from your bowels each day when you are using the herbal laxative. Some people experience what they colorfully describe as a "Ring of Fire" during the Master Cleanse. To be plain about it, inflammation can result from the cayenne pepper and acidic waste being passed from the bowels.

The best remedy is usually to apply coconut oil on the affected area. (Coconut oil is found in health food stores or in the natural foods section of some supermarkets.) Do not use hand cream or lotion on tender tissues because they usually contain chemicals that are severely irritating.

Mix Your Lemonade
—Place 2 tablespoons of freshly squeezed lemon juice into a glass. (Use a
  measuring spoon for accuracy.)
—Add 2 tablespoons of maple syrup.
—Add 1/10 teaspoon of cayenne powder.
—Fill the glass with eight ounces (one full measuring cup) of good-quality
  water.
—Drink up!

Step 5—Start Drinking the Lemonade

The first morning and every other morning of the cleanse, you will
begin to drink the lemonade when you are hungry (normally within
the first hour or two after arising), or, if doing the saltwater bath,
after you begin eliminating the saltwater. Drink six to twelve
glasses of lemonade every day. Drink the lemonade whenever you
are hungry, and try not to let yourself get overly hungry.
Remember that while the Master Cleanse is a simple process, many
people create a little difficulty with it. Therefore, please follow
instructions carefully.

TIP

To measure cayenne for the lemonade: Use a measuring spoon set.
The smallest spoon in the set is usually 1/8 teaspoon; fill it about
three-quarters full. Many people find the cayenne hot at first, so you
may want to begin with less than 1/10 of a teaspoon and work up to the
full amount.

JUICING WITH EASE

Treat yourself to a good-quality electric citrus juicer. Juicers of this
type are far more efficient than hand juicers and will produce more
juice than if you squeeze by hand or utensil into a glass. You may
wish to buy a used juicer in good working order to do your first several Master Cleanses, then move up to a new one of better quality.

Always drink your lemonade fresh. Drink it within ten minutes after you prepare it. Drink it whenever you feel hungry. Start drinking the lemonade about one hour after taking your laxative or after your first elimination of the saltwater bath. Drink six to twelve glasses a day (each mixture amounting to at least ten fluid ounces).

I suggest that, unless you are obese, you consume at least eight glasses of the lemonade mixture each day. I myself often drink twelve glasses a day, and will drink as many as sixteen glasses if I am extremely physically active. I know someone who drank twenty-four to twenty-six glasses a day (that is, two gallons!) while training for a triathlon, and did so for twelve days in a row. If you feel hungry, tired or cold, it is often because you are not drinking enough lemonade.

If the lemonade tastes too sweet or you want to lose weight, you can decrease the maple syrup in each drink by half a tablespoon. If you desire to maintain or gain weight, however, you may add half a tablespoon of maple syrup to each drink.

You can alternate drinking water or herbal tea with the lemonade throughout the day. It is important, however, not to drink too much water and not enough lemonade. Drink water or herbal tea if you feel dehydrated or when the weather is hot. Remember, you must drink at least six glasses of lemonade per day!

Option

For those people who cannot make their lemonade fresh for each drink (e.g., they will be away from home), there is a simple alternative. Mix equal parts of maple syrup and lemon juice as a concentrate into a dark container and keep it cool (a thermos is ideal). Prepare enough concentrate to last as long as you will be away. Whenever you hanker for a glass of lemonade, measure four tablespoons of this concentrate into a glass, add the cayenne pepper and the water, stir and drink. The maple syrup will act as a preservative for the lemon juice, which in turn will help to prevent oxidation of the vitamin C and the enzymes. Note that as soon as you add water, you must drink it—say, within five to ten minutes.

- Never microwave your lemonade! Doing so will destroy many of its valuable enzymes and vitamins and will diminish its effectiveness.
- Follow these simple steps—to the letter!—and you will most likely succeed by having a good, productive Master Cleanse.

PART 2
Master Cleanse Journals

The twelve journals that follow are true stories collected from around the country. While some contributors were documenting their first-ever Master Cleanse, others were reflecting on the experience as seasoned veterans. No matter how many cleanses they'd completed, each person faced their own unique hurdles—thriving, struggling and sometimes even failing to reach their final goal. Every person who attempts the cleanse has a different story to tell, but reading and learning from the accounts of others is undeniably beneficial as you prepare for your own Master Cleanse.

JOURNAL 1

Ella

Day One

I've been anticipating this day for a while now: Day One, the first day of my Master Cleanse. Like the first day at a new school, Day One's approach has been marked with a mix of giddy excitement, nervousness and dread.

But I awoke this morning with a feeling of mild disappointment. Despite the Smooth Move laxative tea I drank the night before, I had not suffered through the dramatic waking-up-in-the-middle-of-the-night-and-sprinting-to-the-bathroom experience I'd heard so much about. I felt quite normal—well, normal except for the fact that I was actually *disappointed* at the normalcy of my bowels. After all, not having to sprint to the bathroom in the middle of the night is usually a good thing.

So I brewed myself another cup of Smooth Move and set about juicing some lemons. My first batch of lemonade went down the drain after I brazenly added extra cayenne pepper to the brew. "I love spicy food!" I thought to myself. "Another pinch or three will only make this lemonade more delicious and exciting!"

Not so. The fact that I like my burritos smothered in Tabasco sauce does *not* mean I am capable of downing a gallon of pepper-water. I should have known—water has the effect of *amplifying* spice, not tamping it down (if you've overdone it on the hot sauce, you're better off calming your screaming taste buds with a glass of milk).

Moments later, as I was coaxing my aching hand muscles to squeeze more lemons (on today's to-do list: BUY A JUICER!), the Smooth Move finally began to take effect. I heard it before I felt it: a rumbling in my stomach so loud that I actually looked over my shoulder to see what had made such a noise. But lo and behold, it was my digestive system, churning and gurgling a warning that I should perhaps remain near a bathroom.

I'd done my research on the cleanse, and I knew the saltwater flush could throw a wrench into any morning plans that did not involve sitting on the toilet. That's why I opted to drink the Smooth Move on the morning of Day One; I thought it might be a, erm, *smoother* experience, a baby step toward the full flushing power of the saltwater. And despite the cacophony in my stomach, the effects of the tea did in fact prove rather painless. By around eleven all rumblings had ceased and I felt able to stray from the vicinity of the bathroom.

As for the lemonade, after the humbling cayenne-pepper-overdose escapade, I found my second batch to be a pleasant-enough concoction. And concocting it made me feel like something of a mad scientist, or like I was six years old again, making "magic potions" out of whatever ingredients my parents permitted me to pillage from the refrigerator.

And finally, speaking of pillaging refrigerators: I'll admit that I am rather hungry. Maybe it's subconsciously fitting that I waited until now to even address hunger in this journal entry; my approach thus far has been to keep busy and avoid downtime in which I might be tempted to eat. It's an avoidance strategy, basically, and not one that I intend to pursue for the entire ten-day cleanse. One of my goals for this experience is to start undoing years and years of food-related bad habits. To really conquer those habits, I'll have to face them, not just distract myself from them. But for today, distraction's good enough. First I just want to prove to myself that I can do it. Then I'll focus on doing it right.

Day Two

Feeling confident of my Smooth Move–proof stomach's ability to handle whatever I toss down the hatch, I took my first slug of this morning's saltwater flush with the same hubris that perhaps possessed me to add extra cayenne pepper to yesterday's lemonade. But they weren't kidding about this "flush" thing. Drinking a quart of saltwater, I quickly learned, is no joking matter.

Well, unless you possess a certain scatological sense of humor. ("Scatological," by the way, is a word that my ever-jesting boyfriend taught me specifically in preparation for this cleanse. Wikipedia reveals: "In medicine and biology, scatology or coprology is the study of feces.")

After a few hearty gulps of the saltwater, I started feeling nauseous. I slowed my pace considerably, taking almost a full twenty minutes to down the whole jug I had prepared. I drank it while juicing a new day's worth of lemons, a process made much easier thanks to my new juicer. While a fancy-schmancy citrus juicer was not quite justifiable on my current budget, I did find myself one of those simple plastic juicers (the ones that look like little sombreros), and it worked great. It kept the pits and pulp out of the lemonade, and didn't subject my hands to such an intense morning workout!

But back to the saltwater flush. Despite my nausea and a feeling of general bloatedness, the flush wasn't as dramatic as I'd heard it would be. In fact, nothing much happened at all—aside from the aforementioned symptoms, I really just had to pee a lot.

A quick Google inquiry yielded some potentially helpful information: Those whose diets are high in meat or dairy often prove a little resistant to flushing. I'm not a big meat eater, but I eat enough cheese to keep quite a number of dairy farms in business, and although I tried to cut down during the week leading up to the fast, I wouldn't be surprised if this was the reason my system was a bit clogged. Instead of downing another quart of saltwater (as some websites suggested), I decided to stick to the official instructions and wait and see if tomorrow's flush would be any more productive.

The nausea from the saltwater lasted a good hour or so. I had to force myself to drink my lemonade. I guess in one sense, the nausea was a blessing—at least I wasn't starving!

By late afternoon, I felt much better. Perhaps because of the saltwater, my periodic trips to the bathroom were not just to pee out the quarts and quarts of lemonade I consumed. Nothing urgent, nothing neon-colored or particularly picturesque, but things were definitely moving through my digestive system.

I started to get hungry around dinnertime. I wondered, though, if I was actually hungry—or if I was reacting to the disruption of an evening ritual that revolves around food. In a (slightly humorous) effort to maintain the ritual and pacify my boyfriend, who was looking forlorn at the dinner table all by himself, I poured my lemonade into a bowl and ate it like soup with a spoon. "See?" I said, "We can still have meals together. . . ."

He looked unconvinced but appreciated the effort. And I think I appreciated it, too—it made the evening feel a little less weird, a little less disrupted.

Day Three

This morning it felt like the cleanse finally "clicked," finally started to kick in. Emotionally, this was what I had been waiting for: an experience of some intensity, the feeling that I was making a major change, embarking on a significant journey.

Physically, well . . . let's just say I finally understood what all the poop jokes were about.

I woke up feeling slightly achy, like I had the beginnings of a mild flu. My throat felt sticky. Hoping to soothe this feeling in my throat, I went straight for the saltwater, drinking it faster than I had the day before. Almost immediately after I drained the jug, I felt that bloated feeling again—only this time, it was accompanied by a rather urgent need to beeline for the toilet. I was eliminating mostly liquid, and a lot of gas. I couldn't help but be reminded of a trip to India a few years ago, when an order of saag paneer from a questionably sanitary restaurant left me in a similar condition.

"At least we don't have a squat toilet," my boyfriend reminded me kindly before leaving for work.

The fact that, as a freelancer, I did not to have to go into any office on this particular Monday was both a blessing and a curse. My boyfriend had been home over the weekend; his presence provided entertainment and general distraction from my days *sans* food. But today I was alone in the house for most of the day, and I found myself yearning to eat. I was hungry, sure—but mostly I found myself wandering in and out of the kitchen, fighting the urge to open the refrigerator as I often do when bored or needing a break from a project. My trips to the kitchen usually provide a certain structure to my days. Mealtimes are markers in the day's progression. Without these markers, I felt very much adrift.

The achy feeling I had woken up with intensified into a moderate headache as the day went on. After about an hour and a half, the effects of the saltwater flush seemed to be under control, and I was able to finish off the day's first batch of lemonade without feeling like it was going straight out the other end. But the headache persisted, and with it I felt a vague sense of anxiousness.

This anxiousness was accompanied by a resurgence of cynicism about the cleanse. I'd read that the transition into cleansing is easier if you first give up certain things: caffeine, alcohol, meat, etc. It had been easy for me to give up those things; I don't drink coffee or soda, I haven't tapped a keg since college, and I was a vegetarian for the first eighteen years of my life, so I'm well-acquainted with alternative sources of protein (Tofurky, anyone?). Still, my transition into cleansing proved much more difficult than a simple dietary shift because what I had to give up was my cynicism.

It's not that I wasn't interested in the cleanse, or that I didn't feel I could believe in it. I was, and I did. But without a certain measure of cynicism, the emotional stakes seemed too high. If I was taking the cleanse lightly, then I could take my failure lightly. But I also felt that if I was taking the cleanse lightly, I was more likely to fail.

It was this paradox that troubled me as I set to juicing another batch of lemons. I think it's important to commit fully to an experience like the Master Cleanse, to "surrender to the process," to abandon the usual doubts and jokes. The first two days were easy, but today I felt tested. My knee-jerk response to this kind of difficulty would be to make a snarky remark about the cleanse, to question its logic and its reasonableness. But I took a few deep breaths, reminded myself of the potential benefits of facing up to such a challenge, and finished juicing my lemons.

By the end of the day, both my physical and emotional state had improved. My headache lessened, and my stomach felt far less fragile than it had in the hours following the saltwater flush. I went for a long evening walk with a friend, and it was nice to get outside, to be reminded of my body's ability to move. It had been a while since I had just walked, not to get anywhere, but simply for the sake of movement.

Day Four

Despite having gone to sleep before midnight last night, I slept until almost eleven today. I woke up with a splitting headache and the same sticky feeling in my throat. I stumbled to the bathroom to brush my teeth, and, in doing so, caught a glimpse of myself in the mirror. I paused mid-brush, mouth agape.

Was it 1998? Was I sixteen again?

No, I didn't look like I had discovered the fountain of youth—or rather, not the fountain of youth that anyone would *want* to discover. What I looked like was someone whose face was breaking out in angry, red, adolescent acne.

A little background on this: I struggled with my complexion as a teenager. My skin was never quite bad enough to merit a prescription solution, but never quite good enough to be cured by your average over-the-counter acne product. When I turned twenty, though, things magically improved—and before this morning, it had been years since I'd experienced anything more than an occasional pimple.

That said, my skin has never been the smooth, invisibly pored, creamy-soft organism that might have held up in a close-up on the cover of *Cosmo*. And so this latest development in the cleansing process, though initially horrifying to behold, was actually kind of exciting. Was this breakout a sign of my body truly cleansing, purging itself of whatever toxins had built up under my skin for all these years?

I washed my face and decided to avoid mirrors for the rest of the day. (Conveniently, I had not planned many social engagements, having assumed that the laxative effects of the cleanse would make me a bad party guest anyway.)

Next it was time for the saltwater flush. Physically, the flush produced similar effects to those of yesterday: a little nausea, a little bloating and a lot of time on the toilet. But visually, the results of all this toilet-time were striking. I was surprised by how much solid matter I was eliminating, given that I hadn't eaten in four days. (Solid matter amid a lot of liquid and gas, but still.) As for the, erm, "matter" itself—it was dark, dark brown, almost black in color, a stark contrast against the more liquidy stuff that was coming out. The liquidy stuff was a veritable rainbow of digestive detritus, with more than a few greenish flecks to remind me, once again, of that ill-fated saag paneer.

My headache refused to relax its grip on my temples for most of the afternoon, and that made things rather unpleasant. I was also getting tired of the lemonade—more than anything, I wanted something *salty* (a slightly ironic craving, perhaps, considering the large quantity of saltwater with which I had begun my morning). It didn't help that my neighbors seemed to be cooking some sort of soy-sauce-oriented feast for dinner.

However, these olfactory tortures became easier to endure when I stepped onto the scale before bed. In four days I had shed almost six pounds! And though I wasn't primarily interested in cleansing for weight loss, there *was* a certain pair of just-a-tad-too-tight blue jeans that I was excited to break out of hibernation.

"Yeah, you *do* look thinner," said my boyfriend cautiously. Then he squinted. "But what's up with your *face?*"

Ah! The breakout. I had almost forgotten about it. I went to sleep with my fingers crossed that it would vanish as quickly as it had arrived.

Day Five

I slept terribly last night. Something was going on with my stomach—hardly a surprising development, but still rather unpleasant. It felt like I had done a saltwater flush before going to bed, which I most certainly had not, and I kept being woken up by stomach cramps. I would go to the bathroom, eliminate a little liquid, and then get back in bed, cramps momentarily relieved, only to be woken up again an hour or so later to repeat the process.

Given my sleepless night, I was torn about whether or not I should still do the saltwater flush. My stomach didn't hurt anymore, but it felt generally unstable. I decided to have a cup of Smooth Move instead of the saltwater, thinking that it would be easier on my stomach. This quickly proved not to be the case.

My cramps came back full force about half an hour after I drank the tea. I wanted to curl up in a ball and wait out the pain—but these Smooth Move cramps were accompanied by a bloated feeling so intense that doubling over to relieve the cramps felt uncomfortable and weird, like trying to curl up after eating a very large meal. I didn't actually *look* bloated—in fact, I managed to observe through the fog of my discomfort that I looked noticeably thinner—but I sure felt it.

The results of the Smooth Move were slow in coming. I felt like a bubble that refused to burst. I wanted someone to come along and deflate me, drain my stomach of whatever was causing the cramping and bloating. My physical discomfort, combined perhaps with my lack of sleep, brought on an emotional crash the likes of which I hadn't experienced since a bad breakup in college. And it didn't help that my skin still looked like a hormonal teenager's.

When the Smooth Move–induced "bubble" finally *did* burst, it was not the relief I had hoped for. To be blunt, pooping hurt. I felt raw and exhausted and ultimately ended up nostalgic for the saltwater flush. Though the Smooth Move may have been easier on my stomach at the beginning of the cleanse, it was much more difficult to take on Day Five, primarily because the effects lasted so much longer. With the saltwater flush, at least I was only tied to the toilet for an hour or so. This round of Smooth Move kept repeating on me for most of the day.

But back to that "emotional crash." I mentioned before that my knee-jerk response to difficulty is to get sarcastic and cynical. While I recognize that this is a defense mechanism, I've always found it easier than admitting that I'm hurt, or vulnerable, or having a rough time. And above all, I am *definitely* not a crier. Today, though, I couldn't summon up the sarcasm necessary to feign fine-ness; when my boyfriend got home from work and asked how I was doing, I promptly burst into tears.

His reaction to this was to recommend that I stop the cleanse: "It's clearly not feeling good anymore," he said, and on the surface, I was tempted to agree with him. I tried to look at myself through my boyfriend's eyes. I had spent the past five days starving myself and making myself poop until it hurt. I had a headache and a stomachache. My skin was breaking out. My tongue felt like it was coated in wet cotton. I was sick of lemonade. I wanted to chew something, anything—even my fingernails, which I stopped biting years ago, were beginning to look appealing again.

But despite all this, I realized, forcing myself to take a deep breath, the cleanse *was* feeling good—just not "good" the way my boyfriend meant it. It felt good because it felt intense. It felt good because I was losing weight. It felt good because it was leading me, slowly but surely, toward a new understanding of how I lived out my days. I was coming to understand the extent to which my days were structured around food, and how that was robbing me of the opportunity to really be in touch with my body. Feeling hungry, I realized, was waking me up from a stupor I didn't even realize I'd been in, one in which I ate "lunch food" for lunch because that was what humans were supposed to do in the afternoons. Without the crutch of mealtimes to lean on, I was gradually learning how to live out fuller days— and that was worth suffering through a few *difficult* days, I told myself before bedding down for much-needed sleep.

Day Six

After a day like yesterday, I needed a good night's sleep. I woke up around ten and felt cautiously, fragilely . . . *clear*. I felt clear. It wasn't like I sat up in bed and a little light bulb went off above my head and I went, *Eureka!* It wasn't that I was having a cleanse-induced epiphany. The best way I can think to describe it is this: Imagine that your whole interior monologue—everything from a more concrete "I wonder what I should have for breakfast" to the more subtle, abstract non-thoughts that dictate your general consciousness—is playing on a kind of brain tape recorder. And in the average stressed-out New Yorker's day-to-day life, this inner tape recorder is set to playback at 2x speed, and at top volume. So you walk around feeling a kind of general panic, even when you're relatively "calm," because everything is happening loud and fast and sometimes even with feedback. Of course, you don't notice how revved up you are because you've gotten used to it.

Now imagine that you wake up one morning and someone has put the tape back to playing at regular speed and turned the volume down to a normal level, freeing the playback of distortion. This is what I felt like—like I was simply okay, and clear, and able to breathe, and enjoy whatever the day had to bring.

I know that sounds intense, and perhaps even a little touchy-feely. But that's how it felt. I even literally, physically felt like my eyes were open a little wider—nothing strained, of course, but it was like the edges of everything had been brought into an ever-so-slightly sharper focus.

It didn't hurt (pun intended) that for the first morning since I'd started the cleanse, my headache was gone. Even the saltwater flush was relatively painless. I drank the water with less effort than usual, sipping it over the morning paper until—*oh look at that!*—it was suddenly gone. Sure, I still would have chosen a cheese omelet over yet another serving of lemonade, but even this craving seemed somehow muted, less urgent, something I could calmly observe instead of frantically experience. I was feeling, in other words, pretty darn Zen.

This was very convenient because I had a busy day of work-related meetings ahead of me. Though I again thanked my lucky stars that I was not doing the cleanse while simultaneously slaving away at a 9-to-5, I did have to marvel at the effects of this "clarity" on my work performance. Again, it's not that there was a dramatic *Eureka!* moment. My clients did not spontaneously offer to pay me double, and I did not miraculously complete the to-do list of overdue or almost-due projects that has been looming over me for the past few weeks. (If the cleanse could produce results like those, I'd never eat again.) I just felt very present, very clear and very capable of tackling the things that needed to be done today.

I wonder if this sense of clarity would have come after any cathartic night, or if it was specifically cleanse-related. Like, what if for some reason I had just let myself have a good cry, then gotten a good night's sleep. Would I still have woken up feeling clear? Perhaps. But I believe the not-eating has a lot to do with it, too, both for physical reasons and because the distraction/routine of food has been effectively slashed from my daily agenda.

Oh, and speaking of clear-ness—my breakout, miraculously, was almost totally cleared up by the time I went to bed tonight! *Weird.*

Day Seven

Something has definitely shifted. Yesterday's feeling of marked clarity has diminished somewhat, but my headache hasn't returned, and my stomach feels, for the first time, stable. The saltwater flush is still producing the same results, but they too are somehow milder; it's really just a lot of liquid coming out, nothing too scary-looking or colorful. I feel like I've reached a plateau of sorts. There's still something Zen about fasting, like some stress I didn't even know I was carrying has ratcheted down a notch.

But a few things are keeping me from feeling fully great:

1. I'm tired. Yesterday I felt very awake, almost hyperfocused; today I feel a bit more sluggish. Maybe part of it is that it's Friday—my one-week cleanse anniversary, and a day on which most people are typically more energized by the promise of the weekend.

2. Speaking of the weekend, a friend of my boyfriend is having a birthday party tonight, and I'm not sure I can go—it just doesn't sound fun, standing around watching people get drunk. And not that standing around *getting* drunk is the be-all end-all of social activities, but still. That's one thing that's been tough about this cleanse—it's rather antisocial. Sure, I can go for walks with friends, but so much of my social life revolves around consumption of one thing or another that it's hard to find ways to go out while on the cleanse. And somehow, "Want to meet up for a drink? You can have a beer while I drink a lemonade concoction that I brought from home in a water bottle, and maybe chase that with some laxative tea" just doesn't sound like a valid way to invite someone to hang out.

3. I have a very weird taste in my mouth. I've had a subtly weird taste in my mouth for a few days, but it only recently intensified to VERY weird. And by "weird" I really mean . . . kind of like I haven't brushed my teeth in a few days. Except I have, and quite thoroughly—but the taste always comes back.

I'd read that some cleansers actually see a whitish coating on their tongues, and that one measure of a toxin-free system is the return of one's tongue to a healthy, uniform pink. My tongue doesn't really look any different than it usually does, but I sure would like to get rid of that taste.

4. For the past two nights now, I've had food dreams. In the first I spent a long time making a sandwich; in the second, I was being served at some sort of fancy Chinese restaurant. In both dreams, I took my first bite of food and then immediately thought, "Oh, shit! I'm on the Master Cleanse! I forgot! Now *everything is ruined!*" And then I woke up and felt immensely relieved that I had not, in fact, caved and eaten something before the end of Day Ten. Nonetheless, the dreams themselves were quite anxiety-producing.

Anyway, perhaps tomorrow I'll regain that pleasant "clear" feeling that I had yesterday. Though the cleanse no longer feels as difficult as it did those first few days, I wouldn't say I felt my best today.

Day Eight

I woke up feeling energetic, and it wasn't too cold out so my boyfriend and I decided to go on one of our "excursions." These excursions are something we started doing when we first met; they basically entail getting on a random subway line, riding it all the way to its terminus, getting off and wandering around, and then coming home. Though we're both native New Yorkers, we've always loved discovering the fringes of our city in this way, and we never fail to be surprised at where we end up.

Anyway, we took the 7 out to Flushing (*no* pun intended!), a neighborhood known for its authentic Chinese food. My boyfriend, who was understandably seduced by the smells wafting out of these restaurants, asked if I thought I could stand sitting with him while he ate some dumplings. To my surprise, I found I could stand it just fine. Although I have not felt very hungry these past few days, I've never stopped being tantalized by food smells. When I smell these smells in other situations, though, I don't sit down at a table filled with the foods producing them. I just distract myself with some other activity. I thought that sitting down with my boyfriend would be somewhat torturous, but actually it proved quite painless. I just didn't particularly want to eat. It was like the act of eating had been removed from my lexicon of responses to seeing or smelling food.

"Impressive," my boyfriend said (not without a slight eye-roll), before reassuring me that his dumplings weren't all that good anyway.

When we got home, I was exhausted, but I felt rejuvenated when I looked in the mirror. (I should note that I've made it a point to avoid excessive mirror-gazing during this cleanse; it just didn't feel productive to constantly be examining my body rather than simply living in it and feeling it.) I had definitely lost a good deal of weight, probably almost ten pounds. I'd been able to tell that I was losing weight by the way my pants fit, but this was the first time I really checked myself out, and . . . well, let's just say I almost whistled at my reflection as it walked by.

My skin, also, was changed. Not only had the breakout vanished; it had vanished without a trace. My skin actually looked smoother than it had looked in a long, long time. Even my boyfriend, who had maintained some of his skepticism after that whole bursting-into-tears-for-no-reason episode, admitted that I looked, to use his word, radiant.

I went to bed wondering about the end of the cleanse, at which I had suddenly almost arrived. I knew I didn't want to go back to my regular eating habits; not only was I enjoying my newly slimmed-down bod and "radiant" complexion, I felt that I had truly made some headway in breaking the wandering-to-the-refrigerator routine that I had followed like an automaton for so many years. I resolved to set some post-cleanse goals for myself tomorrow.

Day Nine

Just when I thought I was totally over the hump of this cleanse, I had a bit of a rough morning with the saltwater flush. I had a lot of cramping, a lot of bloating and a lot of gas—but none of it was productive. Nothing came out of me until almost 2 p.m. (I nearly typed "until almost lunchtime"—maybe I'm not as broken of those habits as I'd like to be after all.) I wondered if I was somehow "empty," if I had flushed out everything that I needed to flush out.

But then 2 p.m. rolled around, and suddenly there was a *lot* coming out. It was very strange. It was all liquidy as usual, but the liquid had a bit more body, a bit more substance. By 3 p.m., I felt great relief, as though I had in fact found that "deflate" button to relieve my bloating and cramping.

Beyond my unpleasant morning, I felt pretty decent, if a little fatigued. It didn't help that it was gray outside for most of the day. I made a point of going for a walk with a friend anyway, and I took it extra slow, marveling once again at the benefits of even this mild exercise. It had the effect of putting me back in my body somehow, bringing my focus back to the positive things I was feeling, rather than the gritty logistics of my morning eliminations (or lack thereof).

One major improvement: That gross taste in my mouth is gone. I still can't *see* any difference in my tongue, but I definitely taste it. This is a relief; the combination of that gross taste and the fact that I'm really pretty sick of the lemonade at this point was making it hard to ensure that I was drinking enough throughout the day.

My friend asked if I was excited for the cleanse to be over the day after tomorrow. I replied that I was excited and nervous. "Why nervous?" she asked. "Afraid you'll have forgotten how to chew?"

Not exactly. I felt nervous, I told her, because the cleanse is an extreme—and I've always struggled with extremes. For example, I used to be a vegan. Veganism worked for me; I felt healthier and lost weight. But when a year of travel forced me to give up my veganism in favor of a more international/flexible diet, I swung all the way back to the other extreme and started eating cheese like there was no tomorrow. It's all or nothing, total sobriety or ten tequila shots, no cigarettes or a pack a day, veganism or cheese…ism. I'm pleased to report that, with the exception of that last one, I've opted for the healthier extreme; I don't smoke or drink because I know that I'm prone to excess.

I think most people tend to equate extremes only with indulgence—ten tequila shots is extreme; sobriety is not. But for me, the ascetic extreme can prove just as dangerous as its hedonistic counterpart. And herein lies the danger of the cleanse: because I've spent the last ten days at the extreme non-consumption end of the spectrum, is it all the more likely that I'll come out of it only to fly back over to the consumption end? Lose ten pounds, gain fifteen? Cleanse my body of toxins, only to retoxify in double-time? If I know that this is my habit—flying from one extreme to the other—then what steps can I take to break it?

Day Ten

Well, it's over—or rather, tomorrow morning it will be over. I feel overwhelmed by the revelations of the past ten days, by the changes that I've observed in my body, by the changes I've integrated into my routine. But before I get all nostalgic and general, let me backtrack a moment to the specifics of today.

I felt great today. I had a full day (or what qualifies for *me* as a full day, anyway) with a number of work meetings, a project deadline and a cousin in town for a visit. I met each of these challenges with energy and focus. It wasn't a return to the high of Day Six; it felt more sustainable, this kind of energy, than did Day Six's rush. Suffice it to say, the fatigue of the past few days was nowhere to be felt. And as for hunger—what's hunger? I actually craved a lemonade at one point today, which is a first for me. I was surprised to find myself going, "Man, I wish I could have just one more serving of that thing I've been consuming exclusively for the past ten days."

So yeah: no headaches, no fatigue, no major stomach issues, no insanely colorful eliminations, no breakouts, no bad taste in my mouth. Just a pleasant energy and focus that persisted throughout the day.

Toward evening, though, I felt myself getting anxious. I still hadn't gotten around to setting those "post-cleanse goals" (as they say, Goal #1: Make List of Goals), and I was feeling anxious not only about whether I'd be able to sustain the healthier practices I'd discovered while cleans-ing, but also whether I'd be able to start eating again, period. I mean, of course I knew that I'd be able to eat—but the idea of it was really unappealing and anxiety-pro-ducing. Would it make me sick? (I hoped not.) Would I go on a Thai food binge? (I really hoped not.) Would it make me feel fantastically energized? (That would be nice. . . .)

There was no way to tell. My boyfriend, at least, would be "relieved." "I'm sick of cooking for one," he said, then hesitated a moment before adding: "And also, we have gone through a *lot* of toilet paper these last ten days."

So about those goals. My temptation is, as usual, toward extremity; I want to become vegan again, or eat all raw, or eat only when the moon is full on Tuesdays and Mercury is aligned with Venus. But I'm resisting that temptation in favor of keeping it simple. My goal is this: I want to pay better attention to my body. What this means is, I want to only eat foods that make me feel good (so much for that Thai food binge). I want to eat only when I'm hungry. And I want to stop eating when I'm full.

That's it! Of course, I didn't start out with any egregious eating habits: I love my leafy greens, I've never been big on junk food, I don't drink coffee. But still, the way I was eating wasn't quite . . . *right*. And so: I'm hoping to use this cleanse as a springboard toward my goal of being able to listen to my body a little better, and pay a little more attention to *how* I eat. I think setting this simpler goal is the first step toward breaking my habit of extremes.

After the Cleanse

Learning to eat again has been a challenging process, but so far I've stuck to my goal and not gone overboard in either direction. I started with orange juice and suffered no negative side effects. On the second day, I had some vegetable broth—a relief, because I was craving salt! Again, no physical issues digesting this "foreign" substance. I did, though, have to fight the impulse to just *eat*: the broth was like a gateway food, which left me hungry (literally and abstractly) for more. But I restrained myself, and I'm glad I did. After a few days of broth, I'm now adding some raw fruits and veggies. These have induced a little bit of stomach trouble, mostly in the form of cramping and bloating, so I'm just trying to drink a lot of water and keep on taking it slow. I haven't gained any weight back yet, and my skin is still looking awesome. As of this epilogue, the idea of that Thai food binge is still sounding unappealing . . . and that, I'd say, is a pretty damn good sign!

Kimberly

This is my first time doing a cleanse. I've never fasted for even a single day in my life.

I'm at one of those pivotal points in life where I need to make some changes. I'm coming to the end of an abusive relationship of nine years and I am re-creating my life. There are a lot of patterns that need to be broken and energies shifted.

I am seeking the sense of accomplishment that comes when you begin *and* finish something. My hope for this cleanse is that it will be a time to reconnect with my body, reflect on how I've treated it and begin to think about how I want to honor it going forward. My lifelong attachment to food as a way to numb my emotions or comfort myself in stressful times is not what I want to pass on to my seven-year-old daughter.

Day One

Age: 40
Weight: 152 lbs.
Waist: 32"
Hips: 38"

Thigh: 24"

8:45 a.m. Okay. It's Day One. After two days at Day Zero, I've moved beyond my hesitancy and have begun this journey. For the last two nights my sleep has been restless due to anxiety about beginning the cleanse. I'm afraid of what emotions will come up as I'm going through this healing purge. I'm also worried I might get sick and be unable to work. My day-to-day financial survival depends on being able-bodied; staying home from work is often not an option. Last night I slept a little better, finally accepting this choice to do the Master Cleanse. I now see this decision as a natural progression on my path to a new life.

10:12 a.m. About fifteen minutes after I drank the last of the saltwater bath, my eliminations began. The stools got progressively looser. About thirty minutes after I drank my first glass of lemonade, my elimination was more diarrhea-like.

2:30 p.m. I'm on my third glass of lemonade and I'm already being haunted by the familiar thoughts of "can I do this—*really* do this—for ten days?" and "I never follow through on anything that takes willpower." I'm feeling hungry. I am reminding myself, as often as I think of it, that I am taking care of myself by doing this cleanse. It's an act of kindness, something I don't often show myself. I usually "treat" myself by giving myself permission to do unhealthy things.

10:20 p.m. It's the end of Day One. Today was my day off work, and Olivia didn't have to go to school, so we stayed in all day. I wasn't sure how much eliminating was going to happen and at what time of day. It was fairly easy to cook for Olivia all day without being tempted to eat. I caught myself a couple of times about to put a bite of something in my mouth. It was a subconscious thing, a habit to snack while I've got my hands on food.

I was cold all day and couldn't warm up. Even with the heater on, my feet just stayed cold. I drank the suggested minimum of six glasses of lemonade and I had to make myself drink that last one. I could've easily gone without it, but I wanted to follow the directions. I was so sick of that damn lemonade by my sixth glass that I can't imagine how I'm going to do this for nine more days!

Tomorrow will be an entirely different day. I'll be out of the house and moving by 7:30 a.m. I'm going to take a laxative pill instead of doing the saltwater bath. I'll just have to hope that when the urge to eliminate strikes me I won't be on the bus.

Day Two

I awoke this morning at 6 a.m. and immediately started trying to figure out how I could change my schedule so I wouldn't have to get out of bed! Keeping Olivia home from school would not be a good choice. After forty minutes of lying in bed, I finally rose. I felt a little queasy and fuzzyheaded. My forehead hurts—I think some stuff may be loosening up in my sinuses.

Drank my first glass of lemonade around 8:30 a.m. after returning home from taking Olivia to school. No elimination yet. I think I'm going to cancel my three-hour shift of cleaning the dance studios this morning. It's a hard choice to make. I feel like I should honor my body's need to rest, yet I feel guilty for not meeting the obligation.

Took a nap at 9:30 a.m. for 2½ hours. Didn't want to get up. I had an intense dream about eliminating! In the

dream I could barely make it to the toilet, and once I
started going, I kept going and going and going.

My first elimination didn't happen until noon today.
Then I had a colonic at 1 p.m., and it was just what I
needed. When my hydrotherapist asked how the cleanse
was going, my initial response was "I have eight days left!"
After feeling so depleted this morning, I was really wishing
I could just push the fast-forward button and be done with
this cleanse. With any process that starts to get hard for
me, my typical reaction is to quit, or at least to spend the
whole time wishing for it to be over. But I intend for this
cleanse to be different. I want to be present with the discomfort and to be observant of myself as I move through
it. I hope to learn something about myself—my patterns—
and use the knowledge I gain to make better choices.

The colonic was a different experience than usual. I
generally eliminate a lot of matter during and right after
the colonic; oftentimes I'm constipated and the process is a
much-needed release. Today I expelled a lot of mucus and
was able to take in a lot of water during the "filling" part.
A couple of hours later I had a little more energy and definitely felt better mentally about the cleanse. My hydrotherapist was so supportive. She gave me a beautiful page of
handwritten affirmations, which I've posted above my desk
at home.

Tonight, instead of a laxative pill, I am going to try the
tea and a castor-oil pack on my belly.

Day Three

The alarm went off at 5:30 a.m. My head hurt slightly
and I was feeling a bit congested. I got out of bed at 5:50,
determined to finish the saltwater flush in less time than
the forty-five minutes it took me to drink it yesterday. I

drank the saltwater within twenty-five minutes. Twice I had to stop drinking to go to the toilet; both times I eliminated mucus. Shortly after that I went two more times, and it was more like diarrhea.

I had my first lemonade at 7 a.m., then went to the toilet again. I was a little nervous about leaving the house to take Olivia to school. I was worried I wouldn't make it there and back on the bus without needing to go again. Fortunately, I made it!

I miss the coffee ritual in the morning, whether it's coffee with the other moms for an hour after dropping the kids at school, or spending an hour alone at my local coffeehouse, reading, drinking my vanilla latte and eating a bagel with butter. This morning I took my laundry to the laundromat and sat in a nearby coffee shop drinking tea. I don't really like tea without some sort of sweetener or a dash of milk or soymilk. I found myself envious of everyone I passed on the street all day who had a coffee cup in his or her hand.

It was an emotionally stressful day with unsettling news—the kind of news that makes me feel like I don't have much control in life. This made me really want my comforting latte. I repeated the message to myself that this cleanse was a conscious choice for my well-being and that the decision was something I had control of.

I felt a little weak today after about 2 p.m. I was ready to take a nap by 4 p.m., but of course I couldn't. First I had to walk all over the city searching for a particular type of light bulb, and then I had to pick Olivia up from school and make dinner. In a way, I like the fact that I still have to prepare and cook food for Olivia every day. It helps me to stay connected to food. I don't feel quite as deprived of food because I'm still handling it and smelling it. Of course, the flip side is I just want a bite! But I know better than to think a bite would be only a bite.

It's funny how Olivia likes to remind me what day I'm on. "Today is Day Three, Mama. Seven days left!" I'll be happier to hear the countdown closer to the end of the ten days.

My self-care ritual last night took a long time, landing me in bed at 11 p.m. I did dry-brushing before my shower, then I soaked in a sea-salt bath. I applied castor-oil packs in bed after drinking my laxative tea. Last night's ritual was very soothing and comforting, but tonight I think I'll do a modified version so as to get to sleep by 9:30.

Nighttime is so much quieter without TV or the computer. I feel a little like I'm falling behind on "things," but I'm trying to hold onto the importance of this time for putting my health and my *self* first—something I rarely do.

Day Four

I began the day with hiccups. I also had them several times yesterday and a couple of times the day before. This is very unusual for me, and I'm wondering why it's happening. The hiccups drive me crazy. At least they don't last long.

My energy seems to be a little more *up* today. It's 1:30 now—let's see if I still feel this way in an hour. Midafternoon is when my energy seems to have dipped the past few days.

My first elimination of the day was after my first glass of lemonade. I've gone about five times today, and the consistency is different. It's a very loose stool that looks like an orangey-brown blob in the bottom of the toilet bowl. No cloudy water.

I have a noticeable feeling in my lower back. It's not really pain—more of a tenderness. I have a history of sciatica, so I typically have a lot of tightness and some pain in this area. As I was riding the bus today, standing up, my body felt lighter, yet at the same time more grounded, with this dull ache in the sacrum.

My left nostril is also feeling tender. I sometimes get this soreness or a polyp in my nose. I usually experience this when I'm on sugar or dairy overload and dehydrated. I'm not drinking much water on this cleanse. I just don't feel like drinking more liquid.

Day Five

I was expecting to wake up each morning ready to bounce out of bed. I've never been a morning person, and I've always attributed that to late-night snacking on sweets or carbs. Now that my body doesn't have to work on digesting while I'm sleeping, I was hoping to pop out of bed in the mornings! Not so. Maybe if I could wake up naturally, without the alarm, I might get that perked-up feeling.

My eliminations this morning have had an urgency that I was hoping would be gone by Day Five. Also, the odor has been very strong the last two days. I'll try the internal saltwater bath again tomorrow morning if I can get someone else to take Olivia to school. For most of this week I've shifted my schedule so that I don't work until noon; however, tomorrow I'll need to leave for work at 9 a.m., so I'll have to leave the comfort zone of my home at the start of the day.

Got a chiropractic adjustment today. The adjustments felt like they were deeper; my body doesn't feel so tight and resistant, so I was able to let go more readily.

I'm hoping to be less scattered in my head and get some things done. I'm not there—still feeling fuzzyheaded or something. It's 4 p.m. and I'm sleepy again.

My lower back felt fine today, but now the achy feeling is in my gut—lower intestines, I guess. The sensation isn't one of cramping, it's just a dull ache, like how muscles feel when they're sore from exercise. It's a little unsettling. I also seem to look paler in the mirror than usual. Probably psychosomatic!

Food smelled good to me today, but I wasn't tempted to eat. The thought crossed my mind, but I really felt resigned to the no-eating thing. I'm starting to feel a bit deprived, though, almost like the choice to do this cleanse was a punishment—not the privilege I initially thought. It's amazing how the ego (master of negative thought patterns that support old habits) bullies its way in and makes me feel bad. I had to fight off the voice in my head that was telling me I'm just going to go back to my old ways after the cleanse.

Why continue? Because I am worthy of a different way of living—a better way of living.

Day Six

I actually woke up before the alarm went off today—before 6 a.m. Wow! Probably because I was anxious about doing as much "cleansing" (i.e., eliminating) as possible before having to leave the house at 9 a.m. I am really preoccupied with this fear of being caught outside my house at an inopportune moment!

Eliminations started halfway through the saltwater flush, and I must have gone five times in that hour! It was more like diarrhea today. After that, I didn't "go" much the rest of the day.

I've been thinking a lot today about the importance of coming up with alternatives to some of my unhealthy habits. I want to make a list of ideas before I'm off the cleanse. A friend asked me today about what I will do when stressful situations arise—she knows that I often use food to help me get through difficult times. I couldn't give a clear answer. What have I been doing the past six days since I haven't had food as a distraction or numbing agent? I don't think I've "done" anything. I'm more self-aware, I guess. And I have a boost of confidence from knowing that I'm sticking to the cleanse.

Reading about parasites today briefly in *The Complete Master Cleanse* piqued my interest in doing a parasite cleanse sometime soon. It's an interesting mindset I find myself in: Now that I've begun cleansing, I want everything bad to leave my body NOW!

Sleep. I need to sleep now. I'm not feeling rested enough through this process.

Day Seven

I didn't take a laxative of any sort this morning. I really need to have a few hours in the morning to be near my toilet, and I just didn't have the time today. I'm not feeling the ache in my intestines and am wondering if that's because I didn't do the laxative. I eliminated two times this morning and only a small amount.

I felt like I had a little more spring in my step today. I think the whites of my eyes look brighter. The soreness in my left nostril is almost completely gone. A polyp never formed—at least not that I could feel. My lower back is feeling good. My whole body feels more fluid, flexible and lighter. My pants are much looser; I'll be interested to see what my weight and measurements are at the end of this.

I keep thinking about parasites potentially being in my body. It was interesting what I read about the connection between parasites in the body and the desire for sugar. I'm such a sugar addict that this certainly makes me wonder if it is a possibility.

Seven days is longer than I thought I could go on the cleanse. My skin seems to be balancing out and becoming less dry. I began spotting this afternoon, as though I'm starting my menstrual cycle, even though I just finished my last period as I began the Master Cleanse. My usual pre-menstrual pimples popped up today also.

Day Eight

Slept in until 8 a.m. today. No school and no work—yay! I decided to do the internal saltwater bath this morning since I had plenty of time to take it easy. I started eliminating about fifteen minutes after finishing the saltwater. This was different from the other times. I usually begin eliminations halfway through the drink. I seem to be gassy after the Smooth Move tea I drank last night. I'm not this way when I take the laxative pill. Finally, after about eight times this morning, there was no more eliminating! Each time it was very watery, like diarrhea, I'm guessing from the saltwater.

I still don't know if I actually started my period or not—not much spotting today.

I got hungry a few times today, which hadn't been the case since the first few days of this cleanse. I was a little grumpy about it. I started craving a lot of my old comfort foods: burritos, pizza, toasted bagels and lattes. Oddly, I'm not craving the sweet things as much as the wheat and dairy foods. Maybe it's just that I am missing the warmth of cooked food in my body and the experience of chewing and tasting a variety of flavors. After eight days of no food, is it really my body having these cravings, or is it my mind?

A client told me of a book, *Eat to Live,* that I think I'm going to get this week to help me reintroduce food to my body in a healthy way.

Today I feel tired and unmotivated to get organized. I was hoping to get a lot of little projects done, but I haven't felt motivated to do much of anything beyond daily tasks. Maybe I'm not drinking enough lemonade, but I can't really imagine drinking any more than I do. I feel full of liquid for most of the day.

Day Nine

It took me over half an hour to drink the saltwater today. Eliminations started one hour after I began the internal salt bath. I eliminated about six times in the first two hours. I also had two lemonades during that time.

I have one day left. Wow! I'm ready to be done with the lemonade. I was really wishing that today were my last day. Olivia was teasing me by trying to trick me into eating. It was funny, but it also made me realize how social eating is for us. We all know that food is a big part of being social in our culture, and on a day-to-day basis it just feels good to share our food with the people we care about.

During this process, I've sheltered myself from my normal socializing. I needed the time and space for introspection, and I frankly found it necessary due to what my body was going through—these haven't exactly been my prettiest moments! Reintegrating into my normal life in two days will be interesting. I'm feeling a bit nervous about it.

I got some things done today and last night. Watching less TV has been good. I really do watch TV and eat as a double-whammy way of escaping my feelings.

My menstrual spotting didn't continue today. It was just an odd one-day thing. My PMS pimple came to a head quickly and was gone. (They usually linger for two or three days.)

I've felt hungry and not so nourished the last two days. It's definitely time to come off the lemonade.

Day Ten

Weight: 142 lbs.

Waist: 30"

Hips: 36"

Thigh: 23"

Didn't eliminate today until after lemonade #2, to which I added a little extra cayenne in hopes of getting things moving.

The last two days of this cleanse I have felt hungry and been really moody and agitated, even angry. Poor Olivia. I've turned into Mommy Dearest. Every time she whines that she's hungry and wants something to eat, I snap at her with, "You're hungry? I haven't eaten for ten days!" Okay. She's seven, and she's not the one who decided I wouldn't eat for ten days. I must be getting impatient knowing that the end is near.

I'm also feeling anxious about the end. I'm really looking forward to food, yet I'm worried about what will happen when I'm left to make choices again. I've made bad decisions for years. How do I trust that I will make good, healthy choices going forward?

This fast has served as an emotional cleanse as well as a physical one. It has been a symbol of a responsible choice. In the past, because I did not honor, respect and value myself, I chose to put myself in a relationship where I was dishonored, disrespected and de-valued by another person. The last ten days have been an exercise in honoring, respecting and valuing me. It wasn't always comfortable. I questioned my motivation and my resolve along the way, but at the end of each day I was proud of myself. Pride is not something I've felt much of in the last decade.

The Master Cleanse has given me the opportunity to cleanse and detoxify my body; the space to assess my eating patterns and think of how I want to create new habits; and most importantly, it's given me a chance to reclaim the self-confidence that has laid dormant in me for years. What a gift!

After the Cleanse

I came off the cleanse fairly gradually the first two days, beginning with orange juice and fruit for most of the first day, ending with a homemade vegetable broth. I went back to a somewhat "normal" diet by the fourth day. I actually had a dinner date the fourth night after coming off the cleanse. The dinner was an Italian meal. It consisted of a glass of red wine and a good-sized portion of pasta. I felt extremely full after this meal and certainly felt slow and lethargic waking up the next day. That next morning I drank a latte and ate half a bagel.

A week after coming off the cleanse, I had an extreme reaction to alcohol. This happened on another dinner date (I think I advise not dating for a month after coming off the cleanse!). I drank too much. Under normal circumstances I would have been able to handle this amount of alcohol, but this time I got extremely intoxicated. It didn't happen right away, but my hangover the next day was one of the worst I have ever experienced. My body was trying desperately to purge the toxins I had put in. I couldn't vomit, but my bowels kept eliminating. I was nauseated and could barely get myself to drink anything, which left me severely dehydrated by the end of the day. My body slowly recovered in the week following this incident.

Aside from this, my food choices have continued to be a combination of old, familiar, not-so-healthy choices, plus some good choices, too. I haven't moved right into a whole new way of eating like I had hoped I would be motivated to do. However, I have been eating a lot more fresh, organic fruits and vegetables every day. I find that I am very conscious of how my body feels after eating certain foods. I have a clearer sense of what foods (and drinks!) I'm reacting to positively and negatively. I am making an effort to not be so harsh in judging myself for the "bad" choices. When I'm ready to completely give certain things up, I will.

I will definitely do this cleanse again and I'm curious about what it will reveal the next time around.

Noel

Day One

I've been experiencing what I think are allergies for the past couple of days, and that's the main reason I decided to do the Master Cleanse. Last night, I woke up a couple of times needing water for the itching in the back of my throat. I can't say for sure what's triggering these allergy symptoms, but I'm hoping the Master Cleanse can help me flush out my system and get rid of them. Losing a little weight wouldn't hurt, either (I'm about ten pounds over my ideal).

Yesterday would've been a better day to start, but I didn't plan ahead and have the tea the night before, so I had to wait until today. I have a friend coming to visit in twelve days, and I want to be back to eating real food when she's here. If I'm going to try for the full ten-day cleanse—which, I have to say, seems almost impossible, so much so that I haven't told anyone I'm attempting it yet— and have ample time to reintegrate good food into my diet, I need to start now.

I definitely need a jump-start on my diet. I've got a trip to New York coming up soon, and I want to fit back into all of the clothes I used to wear when I lived there. While I don't really expect to lose all that much permanent weight through the cleanse, I am hoping it motivates me enough to keep trying for a while after my friend leaves so that I can enjoy my time in the city and feel good about myself.

I am a little concerned about going to my dance classes for the next three days. It will be a real test to get there on time if the saline drink has the effect it supposedly has. But I still want to go—I need the exercise. I am encouraged by the blogs of people who say they worked out while doing the cleanse.

It sounds like the best way to get through this is to not tell many people what you're doing and to avoid tempting situations. I am most concerned about Thursday, which will be Day Five if I make it that far. I'm supposed to go on a boat trip with my girlfriends. On an occasion like this, we would usually have a nice drink, and maybe some french fries, too, but that's going to be out for me. I will have to be content with my lemonade and water.

As I'm typing this, I'm trying to get my first round of the saline drink down. I had no idea that two teaspoons could make a whole quart of water so damn salty. I sort of like salty things, but this is gross. I had this plan of just downing it, to speed up the process, but I think I might throw up if I try to do that. So I am trying to get it down in half an hour. I hope something will happen within an hour after that. I want to know approximately how early I need to drink the saline in order to leave on time for my dance class tomorrow.

. . .

I only managed to get about twenty-four ounces of the saltwater down. I read that some people just drink the tea in the evening and in the morning; maybe that's what I'll have to do. Although I am anxious to try the lemonade, I am going to wait an hour to see if anything happens from the saltwater flush. I don't think I could down much more liquid right now anyway.

. . .

Twenty-four ounces was apparently enough. I just spent the last half hour in the bathroom, beginning about fifteen minutes after that last entry. My stomach hurt for a second and then I knew. If the results are that quick then I will definitely be able to make it to my dance class in the morning, although I'd want to drink some lemonade, too, to get some energy. So far (a whole hour into the cleanse!), everything is going according to plan. I'm not hungry yet, but I don't generally eat a big breakfast, if any, so I probably won't feel like I'm starving until lunchtime.

. . .

The lemonade is spicy! I think I may have accidentally only put in two tablespoons of syrup for two servings of lemonade, but either way, that cayenne is going to kick my butt. I might be particularly sensitive to it right now because my throat is a little sore. I can see now, though, why it might actually be hard to get all of it down in a day.

. . .

I didn't really feel hungry all day. So far, I've just realized how much I eat simply because I think it's time to eat. I did cheat by sucking on a lozenge earlier because my itchy throat was driving me crazy. I realize that this can get the digestive system going again and works against the cleanse, but hopefully it doesn't set me back too far. I'm going to drink another two glasses of lemonade (for a total of six for the day) and then have my tea before bed.

Day Two

Last night I dreamt that I accidentally ate a bite of a hot dog (which is sort of weird since I don't usually eat hot dogs). Then, when I went to throw it away, I was tempted to take another bite, but I didn't. I remember thinking that I was going to continue the cleanse even though I had messed up. I guess I'm pretty proud of my subconscious! When I woke up enough to remember that it was just a dream, I was really excited.

I went to the bathroom almost as soon as I got out of bed; in fact, I think "the urge" may have been what woke me. I don't think I could ever do the cleanse if I was away from home overnight. I have to feel comfy and know that I can run to the toilet if I need to.

I managed to get a little more of the saltwater down this morning—thirty ounces—and I am hoping it will make its way through soon so I'll have time to get ready for dance class. The saltwater flush is definitely the worst part of the Master Cleanse.

I went ahead and made two glasses of the lemonade to take along with me. Last night, I started diluting the lemonade to help get the cayenne down. I figure it's the same as drinking a glass of water afterward and that as long as I am getting the same amount of nutrients, it should be fine.

. . .

The saltwater worked again, within the hour. I finished drinking it at about 8:10 a.m. and was out of the bathroom by 9:10 a.m. So it looks like I'll be able to keep doing the saltwater flush on a daily basis. I am really tempted to just use the tea or nothing at all in the mornings, like some people apparently do, but I guess the whole point is to get the gunk out, and the saltwater flush seems to be the most effective way of doing that. I just hope it gets easier each day. I was thinking that what comes out after the saltwater flush should be a lot cleaner-looking today, but it wasn't; everything was still very yellowy-brown. Apparently, there's a lot more to cleanse.

Dance class felt good today. The only thing bothering me was my runny nose. I'm not sure if that's a result of detoxing or just a coincidence.

I've started checking out the CureZone Master Cleanse forum. It's nice to know that lots of other people out there are doing this. There are a few folks who sound like they've done it quite a few times and really know what they're talking about. I even posted some questions about whether it's okay to dilute the lemonade.

I've already had my six glasses of lemonade for the day, but I'll probably have another two glasses for dinner. Everyone on the forum seems to agree that Days Three through Five are the hardest, so I am gearing up for that. I think if I make it through Day Five (boat trip), I will be able to do all ten. Right now, all I can think about is having french fries with my friend when she gets here. Of course, it would be even better if being on the cleanse convinces me that all I want is veggies.

Day Three

I think I need to try to drink my tea a little later in the evening so that I don't have to wake up and hang out in the bathroom for half an hour in the middle of the night. On the other hand, I sort of like feeling empty when I wake up and being able to go ahead with the saltwater flush. I thought taking both would just result in one big bathroom session, but it turns out there are at least two eliminations every morning.

I drank the saltwater flush warm this morning. Someone on the forum suggested imagining that I was drinking chicken soup. It was still pretty gross, but today is the first day I managed to get it all down, and in record time. I am hoping that getting it down fast means it will exit a little faster, too.

I also saw another suggestion for the saltwater flush that I might try. Basically, you do a super-salty shooter with all the salt dissolved in about a fourth of a cup of water, and then you wash it down with what's left of the thirty-two ounces of water. You can even suck on a lemon afterwards to help with the taste. I may gag, but the woman who said she does it this way gets results in twenty to thirty minutes.

Today's saltwater flush is not working as quickly as it has the past two days, and I am getting a little anxious. At the moment, I just feel like I have a swollen belly.

It's funny what people do to get through the Master Cleanse. One woman suggested putting ten Post-its up on the wall and then taking one down for each day done. I decided to fill in big blocks in an Excel file on my computer instead so I can keep the visual aid to myself. It is actually kind of nice to see that I'm a fifth of the way through and to have the mini-reward of filling in a block each night. With Day Three almost done, I am beginning to think I may make it all ten days, and I know that seeing just one or two glaring white blocks left on the screen will be very rewarding.

. . .

It sounds like maybe I shouldn't dilute the lemonade. Someone on the forum pointed out that it may change the rate of absorption. Others reminded me that the cayenne is needed to speed up the metabolism so I can't skimp on it, either. People have suggested not putting the cayenne in until the last moment, so maybe for the boat trip I'll take a jug of the lemonade and a little bag of the cayenne to add to individual glasses. The lemonade is pretty sweet, so I may start cutting back on the maple syrup a little, maybe 1½ tablespoons instead of the full two, when I don't have a really active day ahead and can spare a few calories.

Day Four

Everything yesterday worked out fine, even going to lunch with the girls after ballet class. I helped my sweetie make dinner last night, and while I was tempted to stick little morsels into my mouth, I caught myself. Now that I made it through Day Three and am officially on what is supposed to be one of the hardest days, I am definitely going for all ten. It would be a shame to come this far and not make it. Plus, I have a million lemons and a lot of maple syrup.

I let the water for the saltwater flush sit overnight so that it was neither too hot nor too cold. This morning, I was able to get the saltwater down in record time—fifteen minutes. I also drank the tea a little later last night so I woke up this morning around 6 a.m. instead of 3 a.m., which was nice. But now half an hour has passed and nothing is happening. Maybe the process slows down as you progress through the cleanse and have less gunk to get out?

. . .

The saltwater flush worked eventually, but it didn't feel great going down or coming out.

I had to go downtown today, which involved smelling and thinking about food a lot. It seemed much harder than yesterday. I mainly noticed how there's food everywhere, most of it unhealthy. I'm still craving junk food. It's not like I'm dreaming of a nice crunchy salad with no dressing. But now that I am almost halfway there, it seems a little easier to resist.

As a treat, I went to see a movie and, even though I rarely indulge in popcorn with the greasy so-called butter they have at the theater, it smelled awfully good today. I think it was especially hard because I didn't bring my lemonade.

My nose is still a little runny and stuffy. I hope this is the detoxing and that it goes away soon. Tomorrow will be a long day otherwise.

Day Five

Well, here we are on hump day. I woke up nice and early so that I could be done with the bathroom before meeting my friends to spend the day on the boat. Having so few calories, I've felt really cold a lot of the time, so some sunshine will be nice today. I'll have to be careful to stay hydrated.

Yesterday, I wound up only drinking six glasses of lemonade. After the sixth glass, I felt full and kind of bloated, and I just wanted to move on to the tea (which, by the way, woke me up around 3 a.m. again). I think I could go with fewer than six glasses a day, even with reduced maple syrup, but I still want to make sure that I get all six down so I have enough calories to keep me moving.

I read on the forum that some people believe any fast based on sugar (like the Master Cleanse) is not good for weight loss. Some people think that all you lose on the Master Cleanse is muscle and that juice fasts are better. That makes me feel bad about not officially exercising yesterday.

I have been feeling nice and light in the mornings before the saltwater flush. This morning, I was tempted to just drink tea and see what happened, but then I felt guilty. It seems to me that if I *can* do the saltwater flush in the morning, I should. So I went ahead and did it again, the shot way, sucking on a lemon wedge right after the shot and before downing the water. I'm torn between going by the book and going by what feels right for my body; the saltwater flush makes me feel pretty terrible at first, and sometimes even after I go to the bathroom I feel bloated, like I'm retaining water. I know that with this cleanse, what feels bad at first may in fact be quite good for you in the long run. I'm drinking some warm water right now to help things along.

I've definitely realized that every day is different on this cleanse. Yesterday, when I couldn't see any change in my figure, I wondered why I was doing this at all, even though I know that expecting a miracle in five days is ridiculous and that losing weight isn't the point of this cleanse. Today, on the other hand, even though I still have a belly and love handles, I got a mental glimpse of how I would like to feel all the time. At least this morning, I can envision the endpoint—the light at the end of the tunnel. Maybe it's because I'm almost halfway through, but now I'm focusing more on the thinner, healthier me that this cleanse is just the first step towards and less on getting through another day of "starving myself."

. . .

The shot method seemed to work just like the regular saltwater flush, not any faster or slower. I bought a generic sea salt, but it sounds like Celtic sea salt might've been a less painful (I can't see how it could be much tastier), although more expensive, choice. By the way, I was amazed at how expensive the maple syrup was and how much more organic lemons cost than regular ones. The cleanse isn't all that expensive when you consider how much I would've spent on food for ten days, but it still stung a little at the checkout.

. . .

The hardest part about being on the boat with my friends today was not having a cocktail, which had more to do with habit than with hunger. Maybe I was a little low-energy today and less talkative, perhaps even a bit moody. I took four glasses worth of lemonade, with the cayenne in a separate baggie, and it worked fine, although the lemonade did not taste as good when it got warm.

. . .

I just tried on some pants to find that they don't fit any better than they did five days ago. I'm still spilling over the top of them, and they still cut into me when I sit. I feel so discouraged right now. There went the optimism I was feeling this morning. I suppose just feeling a little healthier should be worth it, but I would way rather fit into those black slacks that actually used to hang on my hips. I have been avoiding the scale because I don't want to get caught up on pounds, but trying on clothes had the same disappointing effect.

I got my period a full day early today, so that helps me rationalize the fat feeling a little. I hope that's the main cause of the bloating.

Day Six

I made it halfway! This morning I slept in a little, as much as the tea would allow, and did the saltwater flush later than usual. I was worried this change in schedule might throw me off, but it didn't, although the results have been in spurts, literally. Gross. Usually I just have one or two bathroom sessions and I'm done, but I keep feeling the urge today.

So, I think that I will make it the whole ten days. When I first found the forum, Day Six sounded so far away and so wonderful. I was incredibly envious of the people on Day Six, over the hump. Still, I realize that I have another five saltwater flushes ahead of me. People on the forum suggest doing the tea on the tenth night and the salt-water flush one last time on Day Eleven before going onto the OJ. I was glad to read that one woman who has done this before drinks broth and orange juice the first day and then eats whatever healthy food she wants on the next day. That's what I am hoping to do (instead of waiting till the evening of the second day to start eating vegetable soup). I just have to make sure that I only eat when I am hungry and make healthy choices. I don't think I have really lost any weight, and I'm afraid of gaining weight after the cleanse due to my now-slowed metabolism.

I'm going to try to eat a lot of veggies at first and slowly reintegrate meat and dairy, but I will probably try my first alcoholic drink on my second night off the cleanse. I know it's not a great idea—okay, it's a terrible idea—but I also know that I will want to celebrate my friend's arrival. You'd think that after having the willpower not to eat for ten days, I would have the willpower not to drink for a while, especially knowing it could make me sick, but I feel like I won't.

I was glad to get some assurance today on the
forum that a liver cleanse is not absolutely necessary; it's
recommended more for people who do longer cleanses. So I
am not going to worry about it. While I can see myself
doing this once or even twice a year, and while I can see
how getting to Day Ten would convince some people to go
on to Day Fourteen or Twenty-one, I don't think that I
could ever do thirty or forty days. I enjoy social eating too
much. I guess you'd get used to being around "eaters" and
not mind, but I kind of feel like a drag sitting there with
my lemonade.

I'm going to dance class this morning and I'll be interested to see how my body takes that. Maybe it was too
early in the cleanse on Days Two through Four to feel any
major muscle weakness or dizziness. I noticed some aches
in my legs yesterday, and the leg raises I did earlier today
seemed especially hard. I am excited, though, to potentially
work off all the calories I'll be taking in for the day.

I wound up having seven glasses of lemonade yesterday, which is totally allowed, although I've been trying to
avoid more than six in an effort to lose weight. I've also cut
back on maple syrup—I'm using a little less than three
tablespoons in a two-glass batch. The lemonade is fine
without as much syrup, and I am learning to like the
cayenne. I could see how I might want to drink this even
when there's food around.

My nose is still a little runny, but I think it's getting
better. My tongue has been white for a few days, but I
think the coating is getting thinner today. My hair seems to
be a bit stiff, like I've been swimming in saltwater, but I'm
not sure if that's related. My skin is a little sensitive, but
that may be because of my period or from being in the sun
all day yesterday. It sounds like I'm falling apart, but I feel

strangely good. My allergy symptoms seem to have gone away; haven't had an itchy throat the past couple of nights.

It was a little tough today when my sweetie decided to eat McDonald's in the car, totally forgetting that I've been cleansing. It didn't necessarily smell that good; it was just the idea of greasy comfort food that I liked. But walking into the health food store afterward made me realize that I would rather eat there any day.

Day Seven

Today has been okay; same eliminations as usual. I'll be on my own tonight, so I guess I'll just try to get some work done and keep my mind off snacking. Reading the forums has been a good distraction. It is amazing to me that I am on Day Seven; it used to seem like I would never get here, but at the same time I am realizing that I still have four days to go.

I have been feeling so thin in the mornings, it's wonderful. I can definitely see myself using the laxative tea and doing a saltwater flush every once in a while in the future. I can see myself doing a cleanse again, too, but I'd have to consider the timing carefully.

I was feeling a little fuzzy after I finally sat down to start working on the computer, so I went ahead and drank my fifth and sixth glasses for the day, and I put almost the regular amount of maple syrup in them. I don't know why, but today has been particularly hard. I want to walk to the fridge and stick a piece of chicken in my mouth. I feel great; I just miss eating. Sometimes I think hiding out at home and being a hermit is the best way to get through the cleanse. The only problem is that at home, it's just me and the refrigerator, and no one but me would ever know that I cheated. Monday and Tuesday should be better because I will have dance class to take up a chunk of the day.

. . .

Now I am making my tea at 9:45 p.m. I wish it had a little caffeine in it to get me going on this last bit of work.

. . .

In my efforts to spice up the Smooth Move tea, I added some lemon juice, which was suggested on the forum. But I used way too much! I wound up adding about a tablespoon of maple syrup to make it tolerable. Now it tastes like lemon tea and is actually quite yummy. I'm glad I've been cutting back on the maple syrup so that I can justify this.

Day Eight

Well, the tea still did its job with the added lemon and syrup. I have to say that I am amazed by the amount of waste I'm still eliminating this late in the cleanse. I like to think that some of this is stuff that's been stuck inside my digestive system, but that's kind of gross, too.

Today is another day of sitting at home in front of the computer. Hopefully it won't go by too slowly. I feel a little hungry this morning, but in a manageable way; I know the lemonade will be enough.

It's amazing to be on Day Eight. I remember when I started this journal and wrote out all the date subheadings ahead of time. It looked like an endless list of days, but now here I am with only three more days to go. I hope that when I do the cleanse again in the future (I really think I will), this journal will remind me that I did it once and can do it again. It also seems like it could be interesting to compare my first time ever with subsequent cleanses.

I'm not sure that ten days is enough to really change what I want to eat. Don't they say it takes twenty-one consecutive days to break a habit? While I don't really crave bad food or alcohol, I wouldn't turn it down at this point, either.

I read that some people avoid all medications and even go as far as not using toothpaste while on the Master Cleanse because it could stimulate the taste buds and the digestive process. I've been brushing my teeth with a reduced amount of toothpaste, and I'm continuing to take my birth control pills. I hope that doesn't throw things off too much, but it's a necessary evil. I've been on the pill for some time, and I don't want to skip a month and then go back to it. As much as I've been trying to "go by the book," I guess I am making some exceptions.

I promised my mom that I'd go shopping with her today. It might be distressing if I realize that nothing really fits better, but at least I'll be out of the house. My mom hasn't gotten on my case too much about the Master Cleanse. There was a raised eyebrow, and I'm pretty sure she will be checking for any signs of fatigue today, but she's managed not to be too judgmental.

Day Nine

I was a bad girl yesterday. I only drank two glasses of lemonade and not really enough water. I was so busy running around with my mom that by the time I got home it was already time for the tea. But I didn't really feel tired or hungry all day.

Shopping for clothes yesterday was a little disheartening, as expected. Even though I felt good and empty, I was still fitting into bigger sizes than I'd like. I know sizes don't really tell you anything, but they still have an emotional effect. I guess I just feel like a bigger transformation has happened in my body than what actually shows. I wonder if that could be bad thing—feeling healthier than I actually am. Am I going to binge and eat poorly because I feel skinny? I guess as long as I'm not deluding myself and thinking that I'm done, I'm okay. I know weight loss wasn't supposed to be the point of this, but with my allergy symptoms dissipating, I have really become more focused on my overall health, which for me has a lot to do with my weight. When I am thinner, I feel better physically and emotionally, and now that I've gotten this far in the cleanse and know that I have the ability to get back to my ideal weight, I want it now!

Although I have a ways to go on my health and weight goals, I am almost there on the cleanse. This morning was the first time, though, that I wasn't awakened by a need to go to the bathroom. I drank the laxative tea around the usual time last night, but I'm afraid that not drinking enough water yesterday messed me up a little. So even though I haven't eliminated this morning as usual, I am drinking the saltwater right now and hoping it will flush everything out and get me back on track. I have a lot of work today, which should keep my mind off food, but I am going to have to be careful to drink enough lemonade so that I'll have energy. And then I will only have one more day! Making that vegetable soup is going to be very fun! (Not eating the vegetables and sticking to mostly broth is going to be less fun.)

I am ready to eat again, but I'm also worried about not easing back into it properly and having problems eliminating. It sounds like unless you commit to a raw food diet afterward, there could be a lot of problems. Sometimes it seems like it would be easier to just stay on the cleanse than to deal with all the negative effects of food. At the moment, though, I just want the sensation of biting, chewing and swallowing food. I don't necessarily want a big, juicy bacon cheeseburger, but I could go for a nice turkey sandwich or even just yogurt and granola. I don't want to change my diet all that drastically besides portion control. I am not ready to go back to vegetarianism right now (I was a vegetarian for six years and eased into meat about two years ago). I'm just hoping that doing the cleanse even though I'm not about to "go raw" doesn't mean I've messed myself up royally.

Day Ten

Things were back to normal this morning as far as the tea working. I drank my second-to-last saltwater flush and am now waiting for it to work. I have no problems getting it down now. In the end, drinking it at room temperature was the best option for me. Holding my nose and squatting with my back against a wall (both common suggestions) didn't really help much.

I don't think I am as excited as I should be to have made it this far. Part of me is happy to be coming off the cleanse because I think it has made me more irritable than usual. I'm also tired of being so cold! At the same time, I'm still very anxious about eating real food again. I feel so nice and empty, and I don't want that to go away.

Walking through the health food store today wasn't as tempting as I thought it would be; it was just exciting. Rather than squeeze my own juice tomorrow, I went ahead and bought some fresh organic orange juice. This kind is not pasteurized like normal juice. I also bought some saltless dry-lentil curry soup mix that I am going to add to my carrots, potatoes, kidney beans, corn, cabbage and zucchini. I think the spices in the mix are kind of cheating, but I don't want the soup to be too bland since I'll be sharing it with others.

. . .

Tonight has been really hard so far. I am so close and yet so far. My significant other is having chili, which I haven't had for a very long time and which seems so comforting and warm right now. I know that my soup tomorrow will be a treat, but that's twenty-four hours from now. I have a lot to do tomorrow, so I'm going to make myself get through a big chunk of work before I allow myself the pleasure of cutting veggies for the soup.

I'd like to sleep in a bit in the morning, but I don't think that's going to happen; I seem to wake up pretty early these days (not just because of the tea anymore). I am drinking my sixth glass of lemonade right now and will feel so full once I get it all down that I'll definitely have to wait a while before I get to my tea.

Day Eleven

Well, I made it, but just like on Day Nine, my laxative tea doesn't seem to have done its job. I told myself that if I had a good go in the morning, I would skip the saltwater flush, but of course I didn't, so I downed the saltwater and am hoping it does the trick one last time. Then it's on to orange juice and, later tonight, vegetable soup!

I am surprised that I'm not more excited, but maybe that's just because I've realized I'm really limited in what I can eat for a few days. It's not like I can celebrate with a cheeseburger. And while I would still probably rather have a big sandwich with veggies than a greasy burger, I would also want the sandwich to have meat and cheese. There goes the idea that all I will crave is veggies. My love for potatoes and all things starchy hasn't disappeared, either.

Even though I know I've been drinking lemonade for ten days, orange juice sounds very acidic to me. I will definitely dilute it. I *am* really excited to know that soon I won't be freezing all the time. I'm sitting here with a space heater at my feet and a heating pad on my lap, which is pretty pitiful.

. . .

Orange juice is awesome. It tastes SO good. I am having a hard time not gulping it down. I might have some lemonade this afternoon if I run out of orange juice, but maybe not. I want to try to watch my calorie intake (since I can obviously get by on 600 calories a day), and I know I am going to be getting a lot of calories tonight!

Day Twelve

Well, I cheated a bit last night. I made my soup (lentil base, green onions, potatoes, carrots, celery, zucchini, corn, kidney beans and brown rice), and it turned out pretty well. I wasn't even that hungry, but I gulped down almost two full bowls, and I didn't stick to just the broth. I felt really bloated afterward and was mad at myself. I probably stretched my stomach right back out to its giant proportions.

Knowing that some people have trouble getting back to normal eliminations post-cleanse, I drank the tea last night, but I still wasn't ready to go to the bathroom this morning. I had another tea and got things moving, so to speak. So far, despite my fast-tracking, I'm not feeling too hungry or too heavy. I'm looking forward to seeing my friend, being disciplined and figuring out when I can do this again, maybe for a little longer, and definitely when I have more time to ease back into the land of the eating.

JOURNAL 4

Queen Jahneen

I scheduled this cleanse at the beginning of spring because the season symbolizes new beginnings. I want to cleanse what is old out of my life so that I can welcome in the new. Queen Afua, author of *Heal Thyself,* says that when you are having a problem in your life, it is good to fast for the "unblocking" of the situation. Sometimes you have to give up one thing in order to attain another. It would be hard to move new furniture into a room that was already filled with a lot of stuff!

Although I don't really want to set up expectations, I will say that I'd like for some of the truth of who I am, as a spiritual being, to be revealed. I'm hoping to drop a few pounds of spiritual baggage in order to reach higher.

Day One

It seems as though whenever I fast, there is always some sinister free-food giveaway on the first day! Someone is always offering delicious food, and lots of it, somewhere easily accessible. Today was the birthday celebration for the minister of the church I attend, and they were giving away free cake in the parking lot—strawberries and cream.

Everyone was walking around the church with their plates, eating and smiling. I smiled and took a piece—not for me, but for one lucky housemate.

Afterward, I had a business meeting with a friend from church. I told her I was fasting, and she immediately insisted we not go anywhere there was food. I said that I was fine wherever we went, and yet she was adamant. I often debate over whether to tell people I'm fasting. It seems much easier to avoid people for ten days, wear baggy clothes and check in when the fast is over. There are always anti-fasting concerns. I come from a family of healthy-sized people, so their concern would be over my weight loss. I am 5'7" and weigh 130 pounds. I wear a size 5 in jeans. I know that I will only drop a few pounds and that the weight I gain back will be healthier. However, there are only a few people I think should know now: housemates and several others I'll select with care.

Today, although I did not suffer hunger pains, I definitely got used to the idea that a lot of eating is purely psychological. I was standing on a subway platform when I smelled french fries. I took a swig of juice. The hunger went away but the smell lingered, and I still wanted to eat for the "taste bud" pleasure of it. I then went to the flea market, where I noticed everyone eating. I was a bit disappointed that I couldn't join them. I have learned to deal with the first few days of fasting by telling myself that the food I am witnessing is not the last food on the planet and that this is not the last opportunity I will have to eat those particular foods.

I met up with a friend at the market and the quest for food was the first thing she mentioned. I remained silent. We walked around, picking up body and household items; then she said she wasn't so hungry anymore. She agreed to drop me off in downtown Berkeley. On the drive, she pulled out a bag of M&Ms and I almost forgot I was fasting and asked for a few. I didn't, mind you. I wasn't really hungry. I just wanted something in my mouth. I never seem to notice so many people eating as when I am fasting.

Later that day, I met up with another friend to go to a Native American ritual called a sweat. This is a purification ritual similar to the feel of a sauna, done in a special tent called a sweat lodge. There are four "rounds" where hot rocks are brought into the center of the lodge and water is poured over them, creating steam. It gets hot, and for some people this can be very uncomfortable. I was fine and happy to know that I was cleansing.

There was a feast afterward. Fruits, salads, hummus, crackers, black-eyed peas, salmon . . . . The very act of separating myself from everyone else while they are eating can be an issue. However, in this setting, everyone was very accommodating. A few people mentioned that they would be heading to a vision quest in which they would not eat or drink anything for three days!

When I got home, my housemates had prepared turkey burgers. "Are you hungry?" one asked. "No, no." "Are you sure?" "Yes, yes, I'm sure." I have not yet told them about the cleanse and am trying to figure out how to get the least reaction. Soon I will be moving to a new home where my new housemates fast on a regular basis. My present housemates are not the fasting type. I would love to be able to keep it on the down-low, but I figure after a couple of days, they will start to get suspicious.

All in all, Day One was steady Eddie. I ended the day with the laxative tea and a bath.

Day Two

The alarm went off at 6 a.m., like it does every morning; however, today I did not shut it off and roll back over in bed. I got up because I had a heavy feeling in my bladder, heavier than usual. I used the bathroom and tried to lie back down. By 6:38 a.m., there were pains in my stomach. It felt like something was definitely being worked out. I knew instantly that it was the laxative tea.

I think recommending laxative tea as part of the diet is a mistake! Softening stool for an easier bowel movement is one thing. Softening stool to where it feels like a diarrhea attack is quite another! After twisting around uncomfortably for about ten more minutes, I got up and headed to the bathroom. I released loose stool. Uncomfortable! I think the cleansing process should be a bit more gentle. It seems like the tea is too strong and is designed more for people with hard constipation issues rather than for a gentle cleansing and releasing process.

On previous fasts I have taken enemas each day and/or weekly colonics that have helped the process. This is the first time I am doing the cleansing totally from the inside out. This way is definitely different. I was told that this way is better because doing it from the inside out cleanses your small intestines, while enemas and colonics cleanse only the large intestines.

I am lucky in that I am able to work from home a few days a week. Thank goodness this was one of those days! After releasing, I lay back down and went into a deep sleep, the kind of sleep it's not easy to wake up from. Sometimes you sleep lightly and are still aware of your surroundings. That's what I figured would happen since I'd had a pretty good night's sleep. But instead, I slept HARD until about noon. I got up, meditated for fifteen minutes, made a few phone calls and then headed for my computer. I noticed that although today was only Day Two, I felt spiritually lifted, lighter and more peaceful. Work was fine. No major mishaps during the day. I felt a little groggy and sleepy. It was good to be able to stay home on the second day while my body is still adjusting.

I will need to venture out into the world for the next few days, doing business meetings and community outreach. I have a church graduation celebration tomorrow (in which I'll be reciting a poem in front of the whole class), and once again, I will not be able to join my classmates in the potluck dinner. I have a women's group meeting this week that is also potluck. For both events, I will still bring a dish to share, even if I cannot partake! I have a job interview on Thursday, and I think I'll be okay energy-wise. Thursday will be Day Five and things usually get settled by Day Three. I have a nightclub comedy show to attend on Friday, and I may be moving into my new place this weekend! Needless to say, there's a lot going on this week. Although all these activities require energy, I believe I will be fine. It has been my experience with fasting that after the first few days, your energy actually increases. I have learned, however, to keep the juice with me at all times when I am out and about in the world. No leaving it at home, thinking I will be alright for the day. Taking the juice around with you is like wearing your armor.

I realized that I might not be able to wear the nose ring I bought yesterday until the fast is over, as I have been releasing a lot of mucus and blowing my nose frequently. I'm also noticing that I have to be near somewhere I can spit whenever I take a drink of the lemonade. It seems to produce a clear, mucus-like substance, thicker than saliva, but thinner than the mucus that comes up when you have a cold. I need to be by a sink, or some grass or pavement, because it is not something you can swallow. Ick!

As a side note, I am treating this whole cleansing process as a ritual and am wearing mostly white clothing, taking baths with sea salt or Epsom salt, and using a loofah brush.

I still haven't told my housemates . . . and tonight they ordered pizza.

Day Three

I feel like I am having an affair. I am hiding and cleaning up all the evidence—cayenne pepper, lemons—to conceal my fasting from my housemates. They think I refused the pizza last night because I was sad. I did tell them a few days ago not to touch the maple syrup I had bought. One asked why, and I was relieved when the other responded, "She doesn't need a reason. If she says 'don't touch it,' don't touch it!"

My stomach gurgled all night and some this morning. I still feel as though I am cleansing and healing, and that feels good. Although I love fasting, I do miss eating and am chalking up the sacrifice to my health. Sometimes it really feels as though you are missing out on something, and it is best to tell yourself that what you are losing is less valuable than what you are gaining. Without sacrifice, there can be no real progress.

Earlier today I was extremely light-headed, as I did not have enough maple syrup in my drink. I hadn't bought a whole lot of maple syrup ahead of time because I thought the little bit I had would serve me well. Not so. I went to the grocery store to buy more, and by the time I got to the parking lot I was sure I could not finish the fast. I went to the syrup section and they were out of the maple syrup I buy in bulk. For some reason, maple syrup has gone up in price—the only bottles left were at least $30. In the last year I have gotten the same bottle for half that! Also, the only kind they had was grade A! Because of my limited budget, I decided I'd traipse across town to Trader Joe's as I knew their maple syrup was cheaper. I got some store-bought natural juice, as my blood sugar was dropping drastically. I took a swig and decided that I could continue. All I needed to do was get to the maple syrup to add it to my already-prepared drink. At Trader Joe's, the same bottle was $17.99. Cheaper than at the store I just came from, but still more expensive than usual.

I had a meeting at an organization where I'm a production consultant. I have found that it is easier to sip peppermint tea at meetings and dates when fasting. It cuts out the explaining you otherwise have to do if people see you constantly taking a swig of some dark-yellow liquid from a hard plastic container. (Also, I still need to spit after swigs of the lemonade, so it is important that I not have to do that in the middle of a meeting.) Peppermint tea does the trick. It's casual and sociable and available almost anywhere. My blood sugar was adjusted by then, and the meeting went fine. However, I might add that I have never been offered real, cooked food at one of these organizational meetings. I have always been offered tea, cheese and crackers. Today I was offered salad and some sort of Indian rice dish—and they let me know there was plenty of it!

After the meeting, I had a class performance and a graduation potluck at my church. The performance went fine. I felt pretty stable the whole time. Afterward was the potluck. Apple pie, rhubarb pie, brownies, pasta salad, spinach salad, baked chicken, chicken soup, chips, salsa and guacamole. There was more, but that is all I can remember off the top of my head. One of my classmates mentioned that she was on the fast; I told her I was, too. She told another classmate, and he teased her by telling her to go ahead and eat. She said she shouldn't have told him and that he was a bad influence. Then she asked me if I thought it was okay for her to grab a plate. I told her I couldn't break the fast because I had made a commitment, and then she said she would stick with it, too. I left before she did so I don't know how well she held up!

I brought home food for my housemates as a love offering that acted as somewhat of a cover-up—although that was not my intention. "Here's some food from the potluck party we just had" sounded like "Here's some food from the potluck party we just had. I ate already and I am bringing you guys some!" They were gracious, as usual. One admitted he was hungry. I must admit that it felt good to see them happy. Still, it's not like other people can eat for you. That is not where my pleasure came from. It was the *separation* from eating that was pleasurable this day.

Day Four

I woke up this morning feeling refreshed and healed. This is a truly amazing process. I realized that it is usually after Day Three that something natural kicks in that makes it easier to take your mind off food. The first few days, you are drawing on strength and willpower. By Day Four or Five, you definitely feel as though you have conquered something. Today I felt as though I didn't need food at all and barely even needed the Master Cleanse drink. (I have learned not to play with that idea, though. There is no way I would stray too far without the drink, no matter how invincible I'm feeling!) One thing I've noticed about going out and about is that I need to know where the public restrooms are. I also need to remember not to wear super-tight pants with special buttons and a piece of wraparound fabric that makes it really hard to get your pants off when you really, really have to go. Don't ask me how I know.

I had two business meetings, both at cafés. I was very happy that cafés, and not restaurants, were chosen. The first café, however, sold food that they brought to your table. As my associate and I were talking (and I am so glad she did not order food), I noticed the smells from food being delivered to the table beside us. There was a chicken-salad sandwich that I barely had to look at to know what it was, the smell was so powerful. I think my senses have been heightened due to the fast. With my peripheral vision, I could just barely see a large bowl with dark-green vegetables, large pieces of chicken and croutons. I'm not feeling a temptation to eat; however, the smell of food is still affecting me. It's more like, "Wow. Food is beautiful and truly amazing," not "I would do [fill in the blank] to get my hands on some of that!"

This fast has given me a new appreciation for food. It may sound funny, as I have fasted a great deal in my life, the shortest fast being one day and the longest thirty-three days, but I feel like I've finally discovered the glory, the beauty and the awesomeness of food. It is for nourishment *and* pleasure! I don't think I had been enjoying the food that I was eating. I was just scarfing it down. I don't feel like I was really present. I would choose food that I liked, but I wasn't savoring the aroma or even enjoying the preparation. I feel like for most of us, eating is such a mechanical act; we need it for energy and to sustain ourselves. We rarely ever consider the sacredness of it, the beauty of it.

I prepared dinner for my housemates this evening. It was a beautiful and fulfilling experience. Not only did I cook the food, I also went to the grocery store and bought the ingredients. I noticed that a few of the basics—bread, milk and cheese—were dwindling, so I decided to restock the shelves. One of the interesting things about this diet is the suggestion to go vegetarian afterwards. The home I am moving to is a vegetarian household (with the exception of fish) but this household is not. I made my housemates breakfast for dinner. Kosher beef links, cage-free eggs, steamed vegetables and rice. I also bought a natural cinnamon cereal and almond milk. The regular milk was causing upset stomachs in the house. My housemates were so grateful and so focused on the meal that, once again, they didn't notice that I wasn't eating. I had a concert to go to, so I guess that helped. I was cooking and rushing out the door.

At the concert, I saw my friend from class who is also fasting. She said she was still on her fast, but that she was starving! She was on Day Three. She said she wanted to do ten days minimum and two weeks maximum. She fasts about once or twice a year. I generally try to fast one day a week plus three days in a row each month. I told my friend, "It gets easier by the fourth day!" as a truth to give her some hope to hold onto. "I hope so!" was her response.

Day Five

Woke up this morning feeling great. My energy level seems to be balancing. There was an easier feeling, like I didn't even need my juice right away. The first few days it was necessary to have it right next to me at all times! I also would like to say that prayer has helped me a few times when I didn't think I had enough strength to pull through.

Now I understand why the expression "prayer and fasting" combines those two actions in the same sentence.

Until five months ago, I had been eating a mostly vegetarian diet with chicken, fish and turkey thrown in on rare occasions. I was feeling weak, so I went to the doctor and had a blood test done. They told me that I was slightly anemic and needed to get the level of iron in my blood up. They suggested greens, dried fruits, beans and beef. I have been eating greens and beef, as they are the most easily accessible. Eating red meat has been strange and a little uncomfortable—the last time I ate beef was seven years ago! But I could feel the weakness in my body and the need for more balance in my life.

I have seen all the promos for vegetarianism, but I do not believe that our ancestors were crazy, sick or unbalanced due to their meat intake. I do think the way the animals are treated is an issue. And I think that the amount of meat we eat on a daily basis is ridiculous. I have gone in and out of trying to be a vegetarian, but because of my budget, health concerns and life circumstances, I was never able to fully carry it through. I read labels. I buy free-range/cage-free products as often as possible. That might be good enough. After this fast, I will see how I feel. Living in a new home just might do the trick for me, but I am not a "label" guru. I am not into labeling myself or others. If I feel that I need a certain food, I eat it.

Tonight I am starting back on the laxative tea. I cut it out for a couple of days because it said in the original book that if diarrhea started, you should discontinue the tea for a few days, then begin again. I have been increasing my intake of peppermint and chamomile tea to try and balance my bowel movements. Nothing.

Day Six

I am almost thoroughly convinced that the tea is simply designed to make life uncomfortable. I can imagine gremlins in a laboratory laughing about their new laxative formula designed to mess up humans. Last night was *uncomfortable*. I had gas and a bloated feeling in my stomach. I could hardly sleep. I had to sit up several times to burp, and it almost felt like I had indigestion—when I have not eaten in five days!

I still feel full of air. There has been no physical release, although I did some emotional releasing by crying last night. I don't think I cried because of the fast; it hasn't made me particularly emotional. Sometimes I purposely try to make myself cry as emotional work, to heal myself. Actually, it was after the crying that I began to feel discomfort, and I remember thinking that maybe I had gone too far with my "inner work."

The tea has been causing me to cramp all morning. I went to the bathroom two times with no release. The third time, I did release and the stench was . . . wow. I didn't even want to look; I just had to keep flushing.

Now I am in the countdown phase. It's not that I haven't been enjoying the cleansing and the release. I am simply looking forward to having dinner with my friends as a clearer, newer and truer me.

I had to pick up a check today and attend a meeting at my church. I also needed to go out and get a few more lemons. I was hoping that I had released everything. The bad thing about taking the tea at night is the gas, the bloating and the cramping. The bad thing about taking it in the morning is the gas, the bloating and the cramping—and being doubly dependent on public restrooms! I had to pray that I would make it to my destination without too much bodily interference. I got on the train at El Cerrito del Norte; by the time I got to MacArthur station, which is about a ten- to twelve-minute ride, my stomach was gurgling. I didn't know if I should rush off the train and attempt to use the bathroom or try to make it to my stop at 19th Street. I decided to stay on the train and, fortunately, I made it. I got to the building and went up to the fifth-floor bathroom. I was hoping no one was in there. I went in, no one was in there, and I released. After that release, I felt fine. I went to pick up my check and then headed for the church meeting.

At the meeting, there was free food (again!). I decided to tell the folks at church about my fast. They were very supportive. One person mentioned that I was in the home stretch now and asked if I had a lot of energy. I don't. It is reported that many people feel an extra boost toward the end, but I'm not experiencing that. I wouldn't say that my energy is depleted, but I'm releasing a lot during this fast and sleeping is one way my body is healing.

I brought food home to my housemates once again. Today is Friday and I move out on Sunday! It is funny that the people at the house I am moving to know I am fasting and my current housemates still don't.

Day Seven

There may be a chance at me becoming a vegetarian or a pescetarian yet. My housemates and I had the most disgusting conversation about the meat industry today. They are both meat-eaters and eat everything except pork, yet they were able to describe the most disgusting conditions of a slaughterhouse. The conversation began when I talked about wanting to gain weight. Although I fast, I do not like losing weight. I feel that I am small enough already. I know

I'll be able to regain the weight later, but I was trying to get some ideas on how to do so. We talked about potatoes, eggs and grits. Then I said, "Maybe beef would help, too." Bad choice of words. Anyhow, the conversation progressed to nastier and nastier facts about the meat industry and I ended the conversation with, "I think I'll stick with potatoes, eggs and grits." That conversation changed me. All I did was wince and say, "Ewww!" throughout the whole conversation, but now the intention is fish and vegetables all the way! Salmon might help because of the "healthy" fat it contains, and I know there is healthy fat in avocados as well.

The thing about fasting is that it is a resurrection. It forces you to stop doing one thing and to do another. It takes courage and conviction to leave old habits behind, but it is possible to change. The gradual return back to food needs to be done carefully if you want to retain the benefits of all the work you have done on your fast. If you do not take it slow and healthy, you can hurt yourself. I know people who have gone off the fast only to eat candy bars within the first few days. Breaking a fast is just as important as the fast itself. It takes about a week, although you can eat solid foods by day three of ending your fast.

Today I called my mother to talk about family stuff and some minor issues regarding her living situation. Immediately I found myself in the middle of an argument. This was not at all what I was intending, and I couldn't even figure out how it happened. I let my feelings get hurt, and afterward I had a short cry, which I tried to keep quiet from my housemates.

That evening, I agreed to volunteer at a fundraiser with one of my housemates. I took a healthy nap for an hour before the event started at seven. We drove to the venue, and I stayed in the car for a little while as they were setting up. I was waiting to see if they had enough help and might not need me as a server after all. My energy was fine, but I was feeling kind of sad and antisocial. I didn't want to talk to anyone or do anything "chipper." I wanted to get in, do the damn thing and get the hell out of there before everyone started talking "let's go out to another club" madness. It was a benefit comedy show, so at least I could get in some laughs while working.

They worked us to death. Thank God for tips. We were going to tables for orders, putting in orders, waiting for filled orders, adding up tabs, asking for money, making change, checking back in on patrons. This lasted about three hours. I managed to take a ten-minute break, during which I was asked for the third time if I wanted anything to eat. It was a small menu: nachos, hot dogs, chips and dip–type food. Nothing too fancy. I asked for water and went back to the green room. I felt dizzy and overwhelmed. I wanted to go home; I was tired and thoroughly uninterested in serving anymore. I tried to bring this up to my housemate (if he'd known I was fasting, he would have let me off the hook right away). In the end, I stayed and finished the shift, but there was a mix-up and I almost didn't get my tips. By the end of the night I was tired and thoroughly pissed off.

Day Eight

The Master Cleanse formula spoils quickly. I learned this today after leaving a bottle out overnight and thinking it would be okay. It's Easter Sunday, so I got up, got dressed, put the bottle in my bag and went to church. I've been carrying packs of peppermint tea with me in case I need it (you can get free hot water at a doughnut shop!), but today I didn't even have the peppermint tea on me, so I simply relied on air until I could make it home to mix a fresh batch of lemonade.

I am moving into my new home today, and there is a sister circle tonight for Easter dinner. Everybody is cooking: smoked turkey, macaroni and cheese, pound cake with strawberries. Although I am realizing more and more the sacredness of food and feeling sad that I cannot share a meal with members of my community, I am also becoming aware that some of the foods mentioned above might not be so good for my body.

My new household is a group of five adults, and they are all vegetarian. I think this will be a more balanced environment for me. It is a spiritual community and, God willing, it will help me on my path to maintaining a healthy lifestyle. I have found it very hard to maintain a state of balance if the people in my life are not supporting my decision to change.

After I got home from church, I started to pack. I was able to run up and down the stairs and back and forth to the garage with no problem. I listened to music while I washed clothes, washed dishes, vacuumed and got everything in order.

My friend arrived with the truck to start loading. We spent a short amount of time packing the truck with all my things—I had forgotten how much stuff I have! We then drove to my new home, about twenty minutes away. At my new place, we walked up and down those flights of stairs more times than I care to count. But I felt exuberant! There was not a tired bone in my body. I ran upstairs, I ran downstairs, I ran back and forth to the truck and bounced all around. We even made another trip back to my old house to pick up more stuff. I will have to come back tomorrow to pick up a few last things.

I missed the sister circle that evening. My friend and I ended the evening at a café; he had coffee and I had some nice peppermint tea.

Day Nine

Day Nine and happy about it. I do not feel hungry per se, but I am so looking forward to eating. I can tell that I have lost a pound or two by how my jeans fit.

Although I have fasted in the past, never before have I been offered so much free food! I am a little disappointed that I chose to fast at the same time as a dozen spiritual rituals—literally, a dozen feasts!

This is not like other fasts I have done. This fast is definitely moving some energy; it is carrying me over into my new life, my new state of consciousness. All in all, this is a lifestyle change. I am surrounded by vegetarian friends, and I know that now I am going to be going to farmers' markets more often. I may even end up getting a bike! My life has been "green" in some ways, but I can tell now that it is going to get even greener.

After I did an assessment of my new space, I realized that I have a lot of things I don't need. I decided to give away everything that's still at the old house. It's just too much stuff, and as my body starts to feel lighter, I also feel a need to lighten the load of unnecessary possessions I'm carrying.

I am starting to feel hungrier. Maybe it is the anticipation of ending the fast. At 11 p.m. I felt hungry, so I took a swig of the juice to make the feeling go way. After about ten or fifteen minutes I felt an uncomfortable rumbling. It felt the same way as when I drank the tea! At first I thought I could just lie there and wait it out, but I finally had to get up and go. I had diarrhea again!

The next morning I realized that my juice bottle had mold growing inside. There were small bits of mold on the inside of the top of the bottle. I had just been rinsing out my container with water before each new concoction. Maybe it happened the time I left it out overnight.

Day Ten

This is the last day of my fast. I got up feeling hungry and thoroughly ready to end it. I can't do any more! I have had a tough time with this one, although I am grateful for the experience.

I have dropped at least another pound. This is not all that wonderful for me since I'm already thin enough. The first thing I noticed was that my stomach was completely flat after about the third day. Now it looks like if I just did ten sit-ups I would have a six-pack. I am hiding it from others with my baggy clothes. No one has really said anything to me.

Because I started this fast with a Native American sweat ritual, I wanted to end it with a trip to the sauna. Unfortunately, the sauna was closed, but then I was inspired to go to the YMCA and apply for membership. The one thing I didn't do during this fast was exercise. I have meditated daily for fifteen minutes to an hour, but I haven't added exercise into my routine, which might be one of the reasons for my sleepiness.

Ever since I moved into the new house there have been amazing smells from the kitchen. Each housemate is responsible for cooking a dish for the week and, of course, people cook for themselves all the time, too. As I was getting oriented, one of my new housemates was telling me about the delicious vegetarian food she was making that day, and although she also fasts often, she said, "Oh, sorry, I forgot that you aren't eating!" I have been getting sympathy from people during this whole process, even from people who are used to fasting!

Later today, after a meeting at church, I was waiting outside for a ride. I took a swig of juice, forgetting that I needed somewhere to spit. I quickly found a garbage can. When I opened the top, there was an empty bag of Doritos inside, and suddenly I had a craving for Doritos. I do *not* eat Doritos. I think I was attracted to the thought of the cheese! I have heard that when we crave dairy it's because we crave nurturing. Throughout this process, I have been learning how unifying and nurturing the act of eating is. I think that in this society we are self-medicating with the food we eat. Hunger is the symptom of a deeper problem— of being unfulfilled mentally and spiritually. I believe that cleansing, although uncomfortable, can help ease the pain in the long run because it teaches us to separate desire from necessity.

I am already planning my meals for the next two weeks (I have heard it takes two weeks to come off a fast properly). I'm making lunch dates with my vegetarian friends. I am going to need major support while I'm transitioning. I plan to drink fresh-squeezed orange juice for breakfast, eat a large salad and vegetable soup for lunch and another large salad for dinner. I figure I will be on salads and steamed vegetables for two days, and the third day I'll add fruit. I will integrate nuts and seeds by the fourth day. My plan is to eat a 75-percent-vegetarian diet with lots of seasonal fruits and vegetables. I would like to limit the amount of processed foods I eat. I do like sweets, but I'd like to start substituting dried fruits for desserts. I plan to drink more water, do yoga daily and exercise to the point of exhaustion at least three times a week. I will most likely continue to eat fish like salmon and tuna. I will probably continue to eat light dairy products as well, specifically cheese and yogurt.

I feel like my life has completely changed. This fast, along with my new environment, has inspired a totally new outlook on life. I am embracing it and waiting to see how far it takes me.

Susan

Day One

For the past several days I've been trying to mentally prepare myself for the Master Cleanse. I gathered all my ingredients so I'd be able to start this first day on schedule. I even traveled to a second grocery store across town to find grade B maple syrup.

Since my life and work revolve around food, I've told family and friends not to tempt me with fun plans or dinner invitations, and I've warned coworkers about potential mood swings. I thought long and hard about what I wanted for my "last supper" yesterday. In the end it didn't seem worthwhile to buy anything fancy, so I decided to finish off a pot of homemade vegetable soup. The soup also felt like a healthy option for my body.

After the soup, I drank a cup of Smooth Move senna tea, set my alarm for 7 a.m. and the fast began . . . .

I woke up groggy and headed straight to the kitchen to prepare the saltwater flush. I measured two tablespoons of sea salt, funneled it into my water bottle and shook it up with warm water.

The taste made me cringe, but I got it all down in three rounds of chugging. I didn't feel anything from the laxative tea, so I decided to let the saltwater do its thing and went back to bed for another hour.

At 8:15, everything was still in my body. I got up and started making the lemonade. I have an electric juicer, so I washed the lemons and juiced them whole. Juicing the lemons whole makes the lemonade more fibrous. I mixed together the lemon juice, maple syrup and water. (A funnel helped with this step, too.) I tried a sip before adding the cayenne. Mmm. Then I added the cayenne and shook it up. Spicy, but still much nicer than the saltwater flush.

Finally, about an hour and forty minutes after I drank the saltwater, the first round of elimination came full force! Two words: brown, liquid. And again, ten minutes later . . . .

I never felt any sort of cramps from the senna tea, or from the saltwater flush, for that matter. The flushing lasted about an hour and a half, and I was able to leave for work by 10 a.m. and get there without any pit stops.

The day was long and I hit walls for sure. The most difficult aspect was the caffeine withdrawal. I only drink about one cup of coffee a day, but the sluggishness and the painful headache right behind my eyeballs are classic symptoms I recognize from previous experience. Late this afternoon I also noticed a little tremor in my left hand. Yikes.

Now I've nearly gotten through Day One. I've just about finished my lemonade dinner and I feel exhausted but proud of myself for getting through the day and being reasonably productive at work. Time for evening tea . . . .

Day Two

The theme of the day was stomach-gurgling and growling.

This morning I woke up at 8 a.m. and the herbal tea clearly worked from the night before. I didn't have cramps or anything; I just found that the tea seemed to have a natural effect on me, rather than the forceful laxative effect of the saltwater flush.

I got the saltwater flush out of the way as quickly as possible. It seemed to move through my body much faster today. I assume this is because it did such a good job, er, clearing a pathway yesterday. My stomach made noises after I chugged it, and fifteen minutes later I was running for the toilet! The saltwater flush's effects were over in less than two hours. It was just as gross today as it was yesterday. I have to admit, though, it's nice that the flush takes such a small fraction of my day. And I'm able to clear my palate by chasing the saltwater with just one clean sip of water.

Today I was definitely hungry. My stomach growled and gurgled and I sipped the lemonade every time I felt hunger pangs. I think the caffeine withdrawal might have been slightly less today. It's possible that I was simply more focused on food because I was less distracted by my headache. I do still miss the caffeine, though. I'm curious if the bags under my eyes have something to do with caffeine withdrawal. I look pretty haggard. My body doesn't look particularly thin and my stomach actually feels bloated, but I have a feeling that may be due to my menstrual cycle (I'm three days away from my period).

Another noticeable effect is that I'm colder than usual. I have Raynaud's syndrome and my hands, especially my fingertips and toes, lose circulation pretty quickly. I'm used to it and it's not unbearable. Maybe the chill means I'm shedding my fat layer! I treated myself to a few new boxes of herbal teas, and those are helping with the cravings and warming me up quite a bit.

I worked from home today, so I went for a brisk walk late this afternoon just to get out of the house. I'm a runner and pretty active, but I felt a little slower and weaker than usual. The cool spring air was really refreshing, though, and a great distraction. I found it helpful to plan a route that went in the opposite direction of restaurants. The smells of fresh bread and all my favorite foods swirling through the air certainly wouldn't have helped my cause.

I feel pretty exhausted again today, but I'm proud of myself for making it through another day. Focusing on work helps me take my mind off the cleanse, but without the caffeine it's been hard to maintain that focus. Fingers crossed I'll have kicked that addiction by tomorrow.

Day Three

Hooray! I am nearly a third of the way through, and so far, so good. I woke up with a lot more energy, and the bags under my eyes are gone. I assume I'm sleeping a lot better because I've been so exhausted at the end of each day. Dreams are more vivid, too.

My big breakthrough today was the caffeine. I think I'm over it. Don't miss it one bit . . . lie. Actually, I do miss the taste of coffee and my morning ritual of sipping it while I read my e-mails, but herbal tea is a decent replacement.

I feel like I've adjusted a bit more to my morning routine with the saltwater flush. It doesn't taste any better, but I can get it down in a matter of seconds, which makes it bearable. Reminding myself that this is all temporary and I don't have to drink saltwater for the rest of my life helps me deal.

I'm not sure if I brewed the senna tea strong enough last night. Nothing really happened this morning until I did the saltwater flush. I'm also thinking that my PMS might be affecting the senna tea results. I'm still feeling pretty bloated. Seems like after three days of no food, I should feel lighter. Hopefully after I get my period I'll see better results in my body.

I'm really impressed with myself because I was around food all day. This morning I had a work meeting at one of my favorite cafés in the city, and I sipped water and lemonade while my coworkers indulged in their favorite espresso drinks, granola with fresh fruit and a really delicious-looking quiche. Getting through that meeting without my standard cappuccino and croissant was pretty hard, but I was so happy to be feeling good today that it all sort of evened out. My stomach hardly growled at all today, and I think I only actually felt hungry about twice. The lemonade really is pretty tasty—I think I'll keep drinking it after I finish.

Later at work, I had to cut up a warm, greasy loaf of rosemary focaccia, and not even a morsel crossed my lips. My coworkers all commented on how good I looked and how upbeat I seemed, and I know they were serious because I could feel it, too.

This evening, I took another long walk around my neighborhood during what would have been dinnertime. I'm thinking this walking trick might be my new routine to keep mealtimes off my mind. I had a lot of energy for the first part of the walk, but then I just felt like I was moving in slow motion.

Now I'm relaxing with my herbal tea, taking a bath and tucking in early to rest up for Day Four.

Day Four

Today the bad-breath paranoia set in.

Despite some thorough brushing, I noticed a rough-textured film on my teeth and a rotten taste in my mouth all morning. I'd read about the bad breath before, and I finally remembered to take a look at my tongue. Wow. I could see exactly where that bad taste was coming from! My tongue was so white! But I guess that's a good sign.

Nothing was happening from the senna tea this morning, but I did feel quite energetic. I did my saltwater flush routine, and after I felt good and empty, I took a big chug of my lemonade and went for a long morning walk to pick up a tongue scraper and some peppermint tea.

It's interesting how my energy levels fluctuate over the course of the day with the lemonade. Since my only calories are coming from the maple syrup, I feel an immediate burst of energy right after I drink the lemonade, followed by a total loss of energy as soon as I burn the calories. This was evident on my morning walk. It started off strong, but by the time I came home I was very tired, hungry and thirsty—for more lemonade. Then, after a big swig, I felt instantly alive again and got on this crazy spring-cleaning kick!

I dusted, swept, mopped and scrubbed the whole place. After another swig of lemonade, I reorganized my closet and dresser, and I made four bags of clothes and shoes for Goodwill! It's funny. As my body is getting rid of the junk, I have this uncontrollable urge to purge my space of unneeded crap, too. It's almost like I'm on drugs. I feel extremely motivated right now and coffee is like a distant memory.

The other big change I've noticed today is in my skin. I've had problem skin for over ten years, and I knew this cleanse, coupled with my PMS, would surely cause some flare-ups. I realize the breakouts are necessary to purge the toxins, so as inconvenient as they are, they're actually a good sign, just as the white gunk on my tongue is a good sign. I'm just ready to get through it. Hopefully this cleanse will promote some permanent improvements where my skin is concerned.

The good news for today is that I still didn't really miss food. I hung out with kids eating ice-cream sundaes tonight and was perfectly content with my tea. The thought of junk food just doesn't appeal to me right now, but I am looking forward to all the fresh, delicious fruits and vegetables I'll be able to eat after the fast. I'm not quite craving them. I feel okay without them while I'm doing this cleanse for my body, and I have this wonderful sense of calm and patience about it. In other words, I want a big fruit smoothie, but I can wait. Maybe that will be my prize on Day Eleven?

Day Five

Today was long and hard like Day One, except I didn't have the caffeine withdrawal symptoms. I've definitely hit a wall, which is discouraging since I'm just halfway through.

I thought I slept okay last night, but for some reason I have bags under my eyes again and look pretty rough, just as I did the first couple days. I've felt like a slug since I woke up this morning. It's not unlike a bad hangover. I'm not really sure if the senna tea even works because nothing is happening until after the saltwater flush. And after five days of no food, I still feel a little bloated.

The saltwater flush made me gag as usual, but I got through it. Then I made my lemonade too spicy and I think I've been paying for it all day with some kind of crazy heartburn. All the cayenne sort of floated up to the top of my water bottle so I poured the lemonade into a big bowl and tried to scoop out some of the pepper, but it took forever. Ugh! I've only had heartburn once in my life so I'm not sure if that's what this is. It's just this weird cramp right in the center of my chest. I feel like it's too high to be my stomach, but there's a very specific spot deep in the middle of my body that really hurts.

Food hasn't really crossed my mind today. Since it's Sunday, I was able to stay inside and avoid it pretty well. But I am a little curious if this pain is some kind of deeper hunger, like my stomach has reached some stage beyond growling and it's literally begging for something more than lemonade.

Thank goodness I didn't have to go to work today and deal with people. I wouldn't have had the patience and probably would have snapped and gotten in trouble. Instead, I stayed home like a hermit, turned off my phone and curled up on the sofa for three episodes of *Grey's Anatomy*. When a little kid died in one of the episodes, I cried. I wonder if it's emotions from the cleanse, PMS or just that the show was sad?

Later, I pulled myself up and tried going for a walk to boost my energy and mood, but I felt like a zombie. My legs felt like Jell-O, my energy was zapped and overall I just felt pretty depressed. The walk didn't help.

My whole body feels weak and my muscles ache. It almost feels like I'm getting the flu, without the fever, headache or sore throat. I just feel *off*. My skin is still kind of a disaster and my tongue continues to gross me out, and I'm so frustrated because I was really excited about all the energy I had yesterday. I really thought I'd be able to make it through this, but today it's like I've taken a complete 180.

I took a long bath tonight and I'm trying the stupid senna tea one more time. I'm brewing it extra long so hopefully that will help.

Day Six

I'm on Day Six, over halfway through. I'm so impressed with myself for making it this far. I got my period, and today I feel back on track. What a difference that makes!

I feel a hundred percent better than I did yesterday and now I'm even considering continuing the cleanse past Day Ten. No more flu symptoms or pains in my chest at all! I feel good and look more refreshed than yesterday. My skin is still a tad bumpy, but I keep reminding myself that it's for the best.

I'm still moving at a slower pace than usual, but my mind feels sharp, my mood is good and my outlook is very, very positive. It's great motivation for continuing the cleanse. I had no idea this lemonade diet would make me happier, but it really feels like it is.

This morning I woke up and immediately went to the bathroom. Hooray! I think the senna tea is finally working. After that and the saltwater flush, I finally felt thinner. I think with my period, my body is finally letting go of everything. I can tell a huge difference looking in the mirror. My stomach felt a little swollen the first few days, but now I feel like I'm definitely losing weight. I haven't stepped on a scale, but my stomach is flat and I feel lighter when I walk.

I cut back on the cayenne in my lemonade to just a pinch for each bottle, and the pain in my chest wasn't nearly as noticeable.

It's hard to believe that after six days there's still brown stuff coming out of me! Good Lord! That's absolutely disgusting to think of how much toxic funk a person can hold inside their body. It really does make a lot of sense that I feel so much lighter and happier. I believe toxins can seep into mind, body and spirit, so letting them go naturally makes a huge difference on every level.

Today I got back on a cleaning rampage and spent my day off doing an even deeper clean of cracks and crevices. I'd consider myself a fairly tidy person, but this neat-freak quality is out of character. I hope it lasts!

It would be a lie to say that food has made a complete departure from my mind. It hasn't. But I've hidden all my food magazines and have nothing in my refrigerator so I think I'm distracting myself pretty well. The stomach growling and hunger feel completely gone. I am still excited at the prospect of eating fruits and vegetables again, and sushi sounds really wonderful right now. Overall, my body seems to be craving fresh and clean foods, just as it wants to live in a fresh, clean space.

Time for senna tea and bed. Every night I find myself utterly exhausted, but I'm confident I can make it through this whole thing.

Day Seven

After a long weekend, I went to work today and raved to my coworkers about how good I feel. I'm still feeling light and carefree, and my energy levels are pretty high, which continues to surprise me. I was told that I "look a zillion times better than on Day One" and that my eyes look especially clear. It's wonderful that my coworkers are supporting me through this (and not eating any of my favorite foods in front of me).

The only troubling part of my day—besides drinking that foul saltwater flush—is this pain in my stomach. It's back in full force and it's right between my lower ribs, centered deep inside. It feels like a cross between heartburn and some sort of cramp. I vaguely felt it yesterday, but at this moment it's pretty full-on. I think it's like a stage beyond hunger. My stomach growled for so long and it's like the noise wasn't heard because I never ate, so instead of growling it's yelling at me in the form of this terrible ache. I don't feel completely miserable, but it does hurt to walk and breathe. I'd be a whole lot happier if this went away by tomorrow.

Despite this, my mood is still pretty good. I found myself getting impatient and short with the handful of people I encountered on Sunday (Day Five), but for the most part, I feel like a happier person on this cleanse. I also still really like the lemonade. I sort of assumed I'd be burnt out on it by now, but after I cut back on the cayenne quite a bit I'm really liking it.

My skin is all cleared up and my tongue film seems more manageable. I wonder if Day Five was just a big toxic hump and I'm in the homestretch?

The only other thing to note is the effect of the senna tea. It's interesting that it produces a different, er, type of elimination. It seems to be working for me finally, now that I got my period, but it works in such a different way from the saltwater flush. Just like on Day Two, it's sort of like clockwork. I drink it, go to bed, sleep well, wake up to my alarm and boom. It works, but the eliminations are so different in speed, texture, color and smell than the saltwater flush. At this point the saltwater flush shoots this straight liquid, with a brownish hue, out of my body at lightning speed, while the senna tea produces more solid,

SUPER STINKY waste in a smaller amount and at a sort of normal speed. (That's probably more detail than anybody wants to read. Sorry!)

It's pretty amazing that after seven days there's still solid matter coming out of my body. More motivation to continue.

Day Eight

It's Day Eight and today I'm feeling ready to be done again. I'm not a hundred percent miserable, and I don't feel like I've hit a major wall like I did on Day Five, but my heartburn/cramp issue came back again today around 5 p.m. and at this moment it's incredibly uncomfortable.

My day started off well. I got up early and did my salt-water flush routine right after the senna tea, which again worked just like clockwork. I've noticed the saltwater taking longer to get down because my stomach is shrinking. I can't chug it like I used to, which is unfortunate, because slow sipping just magnifies the terrible experience. Anyway, somehow I got through it and by the time I left for work, I was all empty but full of energy.

My acne flare-up is completely gone and I've been told that I'm glowing. My hair feels really healthy and I'm admiring my shrinking body more and more, but I am missing food in my life. A lot.

I miss the ritual of sharing a meal with people. I miss the taste of cool, briny oysters and the comfort of a warm coffee in the morning. (And I think this pain is my body telling me that my stomach misses those things, too.) Generally I spend a pretty big chunk of my day thinking about my next meal. Food makes my life so much brighter. It's a real adjustment taking the focus off it.

The silver lining of any pain, though, is that I know from now on I'll be honoring my body even more than I did before I started this cleanse. I've always been a pretty conscientious eater, but feeling the lightness in my body and happiness in my spirit as a direct result of this detox makes me want to work hard to carry that knowledge and experience with me.

I'm not a vegetarian, but the majority of my diet is vegetables. With all the fresh-food cravings I've been having, I wonder if my body is going to demand a raw food diet. I feel like my senses are heightened and I'm so much more in tune with what my body needs. Specifically, I'm craving Granny Smith apples, tuna sashimi, brown rice and mangoes. I can only assume that each of those cravings represents one of the nutrients my body needs most.

I did some research on this stomach thing and I'm pretty sure it's heartburn or acid reflux. I think taking an antacid would be cheating, but I may try some a tea with apple cider vinegar tomorrow. I feel like I can barely move and breathing still hurts. Today feels like the worst it's been, which worries me because I still have two more days to go! I think I also may lay off the cayenne completely tomorrow. I just have to get through this and I'm pretty sure the spicy pepper is aggravating it.

For now, a bath and tea.

Day Nine

I'm still in awe that I haven't eaten in nine days and relieved that I'm feeling much better tonight. I'm really almost done with a ten-day cleanse! Unbelievable! Despite the heartburn, I'm absolutely sure I can get through this. I'm in the homestretch now, but whatever thoughts I was having about continuing past Day Ten have ceased. I'll be ready to eat in twenty-four hours for sure.

I slept really well last night, as I have throughout the whole detox, but I woke up with the same severe heartburn pain that I had yesterday. Of course I worried that today was going to be long and miserable, that the pain would only get worse. Thankfully, I was wrong.

The saltwater flush has been getting harder and harder to swallow. I can't chug it at all anymore, my stomach has shrunk and this morning it took me five or six big gulps to get it all down. It continues to give me goose bumps.

The saltwater eliminations seemed to take a bit longer today. I was working at home, so it was fine, but for some reason it felt like there was just a lot of liquid moving through me; if I'd needed to leave the house before noon it could have been an issue. I also noticed the stuff coming out was more mucusy and slimy than it's been. The first elimination was almost all dark-brown liquid, then by the fourth or fifth time, it was pure slime.

I made the lemonade a lot milder today, with just a small pinch of cayenne, to help with the heartburn. I also made myself a little apple-cider-vinegar elixir. I happened to have a bottle of organic, unfiltered apple cider vinegar, so I added a few tablespoons to a mug of hot water and sipped on that throughout the morning. I drank a lot of herbal tea throughout the day, in between big gulps of lemonade, and I took a nice long soak in the tub this afternoon. I think the combination of all these things soothed the heartburn significantly.

Energy levels were still running really high. In an effort to detox my space, I finally sold a sofa that I've been trying to get rid of on Craigslist for ages. Then in all my excitement about finally getting that piece out of my house, I rearranged my whole living room in an hour!

I barely thought about food today. I had a lot of work to do and was able to focus on that (in between spurts of apartment cleaning!). My mind feels really sharp. I had warned coworkers that I might be spacey and forgetful, but I haven't had issues with that at all. I'm on point more than ever.

Tonight I'm double-brewing the senna tea as a final hardcore flush before I finish. If tomorrow's anything like today was, there's still funk in my body that needs to go and I want to get every last bit of it.

Day Ten

Cheers to me! My final day started off a bit rough, but I made it.

Last night I drank two strong cups of senna tea before going to bed. My thinking was that I could end on a really strong note and get as much junk out of body as possible before it's over. This whole time the tea has been pretty easy. I'd drink a full cup at night, get a great night's sleep, then wake up naturally at 7 or 8 a.m. ready to go.

This time I learned my lesson. The double brew really hit me hard! It definitely wasn't as full-on as the saltwater flush, but I did wake up around 4 a.m. and had to race to the bathroom with severe stomach cramps. It continued for another hour, all before the sun came up!

I was so excited to be finished that the rest of the day went well. I officially woke up several hours later and shook up my salty laxative drink for the last time. I think getting that final liter down was the most satisfying part of my day.

Later, at work, I had several important meetings that I'd been apprehensive about all week. I wondered how the detox (especially being on Day Ten) would affect my performance, but everything went wonderfully. I really feel like I was more confident, solid and sharp today than I've ever been at work, and all of that came from living on no food or caffeine for ten days!

As for food, it's definitely back on my mind. For the past few nights I've been lighting candles throughout my house, and I'm finding the aromas more soothing than usual. Similarly, at work, food smells seem more powerful than they used to. I wonder if the detox actually heightens my sense of smell, or if it's just the hunger?

Even though I'm ready to be done with the saltwater flush and detox program, I am nervous about eating. I've read up on the post-cleanse pretty extensively and I've stocked up on oranges and grapefruits. I'm gearing up for the next two days with lots of juicing and a visit to the raw food booth at the farmers' market tomorrow. My plan is to ease back into food and stay near a toilet. I also think I'll keep drinking the lemonade, at least over the weekend. It's that good.

My body feels better than it ever has before. I've definitely lost weight. My stomach is flat and all of the initial PMS bloating is completely gone. I think my face is thinner, too, and I'm satisfied with how my skin's looking right now.

The mental, emotional and physical benefits are crystal clear (not to mention how fantastic my apartment is looking right now!). And now that I've made it through ten days, I know I can do it again. I think I'll try it in the fall and maybe shoot for two weeks next time. Now I'm going to sign off and go to bed dreaming of the bowl of steamed rice and the mango smoothie that I hope to consume tomorrow. I can hardly wait.

Nalea

Day One

I started doing the Master Cleanse every few months while attending college in Hawaii. My skin was breaking out in acne because of the humidity there, and I had tried painful chemical peels to no avail. The Master Cleanse, in conjunction with dietary changes and regular exercise, helped clear up my skin.

Not only did the Master Cleanse take care of my blemishes, it also helped me gain focus in my life. Now I cleanse when I am losing motivation with my exercise regimen or failing to meet personal and work-related commitments.

Typically I try to clear my schedule when I am taking the cleanse. This week is busier than usual, but I think I will manage. Last night I took the herbal laxative, which I have not included in the cleanse before. I was hesitant about this because I knew I would have to work today, but it really helped to clean out my system. I did have more bowel movements than usual, which was rather embarrassing since the office I work in has a coed bathroom.

I am feeling optimistic this time. My energy is up—considering I haven't eaten anything today. I have had the giggles all day (maybe this is delirium brought on from not eating).

Throughout the cleanse, I will be doing breathing exercises I learned in aikido class. It's nothing too complicated; it just helps me concentrate on breathing correctly—pushing my abdomen out when I inhale and vice versa.

I briefly considered going for a run today. In college, I used to exercise while doing the cleanse, but I never cleansed for more than seven days. Exercise is not going to happen this time. My sister is visiting from Texas so I have to entertain her and maintain an unrealistic level of cleanliness in my apartment that only exists when visitors come. The tea gives me energy, but with all the other things going on right now, I don't feel up for a jog.

The first day of a cleanse is never too difficult for me. But today I let my sister use my car. She picked me up from work with the bumper hanging off. Did she think I wouldn't notice? Not eating anything all day is hard enough without having to deal with a mini-crisis. Surprisingly, I did not overreact. "How did my bumper fall off?" I asked calmly. She pretended not to realize the right side of the bumper had fallen off. I took a swig of my tea and felt mildly comforted by the cayenne pepper, which warmed my belly. Should I wait until after the cleanse to file an insurance claim? Ugh, nine more days.

Day Two

I have asked my friends to stop talking about my cleanse. I find it easier that way, though it is still painful to watch them devour greasy hamburgers and fries while I drink my tea. We went to a late lunch at Canter's, a Jewish deli, and I really wanted a bite of potato pancakes. Then there were the pastries in the front. God, chocolate never looked so good.

My boyfriend keeps offering me food, forgetting that I am doing the cleanse. God, he eats a lot, and he never seems to gain weight. Fortunately, my sister is training for a jiujitsu competition and needs to lose weight to fight in the featherweight category. So we are starving, er, cleansing together. At least she gets to eat salmon and vegetables for dinner. Instead, I watched *Tropic Thunder* on DVD and made a fresh batch of lemonade.

I like seeing all the pretty yellow lemons on my countertop. I had to scold my boyfriend for using some of my Master Cleanse–approved lemons for his tea. He also enjoys juggling my lemons while I make tea—this is not a sexual innuendo. As a handy household aside: Lemon rinds quickly freshen and deodorize a garbage disposal.

My sister and I got into an argument today about racism in the United States. As the debate heated up, my sister insisted that I was being temperamental because I hadn't eaten anything. To be honest, I am not feeling hungry yet—except when I'm forced to "go out to eat" with others. It is challenging to stay focused on my cleanse while having to play host and chauffeur to my sister. Ideally I would have cleared my schedule to do the cleanse, but that was not possible this time.

The first three days of my cleanse are never too difficult, but I am reminded of how much I eat socially, especially when relatives are visiting. "I'll show you how to make this Cajun dish," my sister said earlier today. (Lately she has been adamant about teaching me to cook.) I suggested a manicure and pedicure instead. I chose pink polish and she picked some gaudy neon shade. It turned out to be a great way to get my mind off the cleanse for a bit. But then my sister made some fish dish with garlic this evening, and I swore I could taste the garlic in the air. Perhaps I am hungrier than I realize. One activity that helps deter my cravings is to buy spices and other food items I can eat when I am done with the cleanse.

The scale in my bathroom shows that I have lost about a pound. I have been drinking more water than I probably should, and I chewed a couple pieces of gum today. Is that cheating? I am not quite sure. Either the tea or the lack of food is making my breath funky (or perhaps there is a better explanation for it that I am not aware of). This only made me hungrier to chew the gum. Note to self: No more gum until the final day.

Day Three

I am growing increasingly irritable. It is a challenge to remain composed enough to deal with normal day-to-day issues. I wish I was a great yogi and could be incredibly tranquil right now, but I am starting to crave food. I cannot endure another interminable phone conversation about how my mother's coworker smells like onions, especially when I am hankering for some stir-fried onions. (Garlic, onions and mushrooms are at the top of my food wish list.) "Remember to breathe," I have to say to myself. I have been closing my eyes and listening to my breathing. It helps curb my tension.

I tried to exercise today, but I got to the gym and realized I left my shoes at home. Perhaps I did that on purpose. It was probably for the best since I was feeling low on energy today.

Luckily, it was a really pretty day—at least for Los Angeles. But I was not able to shirk my work-related obligations. Perhaps that is why I'm feeling slightly tense. At least I mostly work from home. After drinking some ice-cold water, I took a long bath, which soothed my irritability. I took a little power nap after my bath. My sister visited a friend today in Beverly Hills so I got a much-needed break from tour-guide responsibilities.

This morning I put too much cayenne pepper in the lemonade, which actually served to temporarily minimize my hunger pangs. I really like how the pepper warms my stomach. My boyfriend accidentally drank my tea today. It was really funny. He immediately spat it out in the sink and told me not to drink it, calling it poison. I am used to the taste and it doesn't bother me anymore.

On the plus side, my boyfriend has been complimenting me on my skin. I have started to notice that my complexion is looking really healthy. However, a little pimple popped up today on my jaw. Perhaps the blemish is from the toxins coming out. My skin smells like garlic, but it may just be from chopping garlic last night for my sister's dinner. I thought preparing food and mincing garlic would help curb my appetite, but it did the opposite.

Every evening I have been weighing myself. Mr. Scale shows that I have lost one and a half pounds, which helped to give me added inspiration. Seven more days!

My digestive system is rather funky today. Everything that comes out is watery. I am also getting the sniffles. Usually I do not get sick on the Master Cleanse. On other cleanses I have stopped midway through because I started feeling really nauseous. In this case, I think I might just be getting a little cold. I wish I could eat an orange or two.

My pretty bowl of yellow lemons is starting to dwindle, reminding me that I am moving along on my ten-day commitment. Hopefully tomorrow my sinuses will clear up.

Day Four

I am probably sick. Yesterday's sniffles seem to have evolved into a full-blown sinus infection—at least that's my unprofessional self-diagnosis. I wanted to stay home today instead of going in to the office, but that was not possible so I schlepped my tea and Kleenex to work.

It was a struggle to concentrate today, especially since I'm feeling under the weather. I spent a lot of time staring at the computer screen. No one at work knows that I am cleansing. I've found that it is better not to tell coworkers. They usually have a lot of inane questions and become skeptical of my work performance (as they should). The last time I told a coworker, I ended up breaking my cleanse halfway through because she insisted that I eat a banana. After the banana I binged on tacos.

My stomach is still uneasy. I am visiting the bathroom more than usual, which tends to raise some eyebrows at work. I made the mistake of not drinking enough tea today, which only served to make me feel worse. I made the tea in bulk and it was not fresh, so it started to taste rather nasty midday. I know it is best to drink the tea fresh, but sometimes that just isn't practical. At least tomorrow I can drink all the fresh lemonade I want.

When I got home from work, I took a long bath and did some breathing exercises. The breathing really takes the edge off. I also did some stretching, which made me feel relaxed.

My sister flies back to Austin tomorrow, so this evening we went out for drinks at an outdoor pub. God, a glass of wine would have been nice. But I knew what alcohol would do to my system after cleansing for days. I'm already a lightweight when it comes to alcohol, but on an empty stomach, wine would have knocked me out.

It is really not much fun to be the designated driver—those public service announcements are misleading. My mind wandered as I watched my friends drink up a storm. I started thinking about how hilarious it would be if the bouncer checked my purse and found a plastic bottle of warm red tea. Maybe I am delirious from not eating and it wouldn't really have been all that funny.

I didn't have as many food cravings today, though soup would have been a nice lunch. Although I am not really feeling hungry, I have developed a habit of awkwardly staring at people while they eat. I feel like an untrained puppy begging for food at the dinner table.

My daily weigh-in showed that I lost three and a half pounds since starting the cleanse! My skin is really glowing, too. Some of the discoloration on my cheeks is fading and I noticed my nails seem to be getting stronger, but perhaps it's just my imagination.

Day Five

My energy is back! Although I still have the sniffles, I am feeling invigorated. My confidence is surging; I know I can successfully finish the cleanse. If I complete this cleanse, it will be the longest period I've gone on drinking the lemonade.

My sister headed back home this morning. When we said goodbye, she unconvincingly promised to pay for my bumper, which is still dangling from my poor car. That is one check that will probably never be signed or delivered. It was fun having her here, but entertaining company while cleansing can be difficult.

Today I concentrated on getting healthy again. In an effort to clear up my sinus congestion, I slathered a healthy dose of vapor rub on my chest. It worked—I feel slightly better. I also did some light exercise today because I was feeling good. I jogged around the track for about thirty minutes. I even squeezed in a tanning session after work. (I hope this is within the guidelines of the Master Cleanse. Is it okay to soak up UV rays while you're cleansing? It is probably not recommended, but I needed to do something nice for myself.)

When I weighed myself today I found that I've lost four pounds! It could soon be time to dust off my skinny jeans. My body feels lighter and I notice my legs are slimmer. My face is looking thinner, too.

Of course I am hungry and starting to get bored of drinking tea for breakfast, lunch and dinner. I've started watching random cooking shows, which is kind of like eating vicariously. My boyfriend keeps asking me if I want to eat with him, which really frustrates me. He knows I am cleansing. Tonight I watched enviously as he devoured a juicy steak for dinner. He even started licking the plate! I think he is getting sick of watching me cleanse. I am also PMS-ing, so I might be overreacting.

Since I haven't eaten anything in a few days, my breath is noticeably funkier. My body odor hasn't really changed at all. My digestive system is not as bothersome today, but nothing is really solid. I am starting to have cramps, but that could be because I'm expecting my period soon. If the cramps don't diminish, I will know the pain is from the herbal laxative. Then I will switch to the saltwater flush.

I just realized that I am at the midpoint of the cleanse. Geez, I was thinking I had three days left. Maybe some breathing exercises are in order.

Day Six

I think I'm transforming into a hound dog. Cleansing has caused me to develop a bionic sense of smell. Despite my stuffy nose, I am now capable of smelling fast-food restaurants blocks away. If someone is smoking in the courtyard outside my house, I can almost identify the brand of cigarette.

Plans for my first meal are already underway. I am thinking Indian curry with brown rice. I hope to ease off the cleanse with vegetables and fruit. Right now I am craving eggplant and onions.

Lately I have taken to opening the refrigerator and simply staring. I should have had more tea today instead of drinking all that water. I have been gnawing on crushed ice because it makes me feel like I am chewing food. My only comfort is Mr. Scale, who has not let me down yet. I've lost a whopping seven pounds!

My irritability has returned. Today I got into a ridiculous semi-argument with a coworker about pronouns. I am having wicked stomach cramps, too. Hello, PMS! Actually I'm still not sure if it's PMS or side effects from the laxative. My bowel movements seem unusually frequent. Everything is starting to hurt.

My energy is waning. Usually I would end my cleanse tomorrow—I have never done it longer than seven days. This is truly a mental challenge as much as a physical one. Interestingly, I am having small bursts of clarity. For instance, at the office today, after what would have been my lunch break, I started working nonstop without daydreaming about food. I know this sounds ridiculous, but it was a big step.

The good news is that I'm sleeping soundly. Prior to starting the cleanse, I had to take two Tylenol PMs every night. I really hate depending on sleeping pills. But now my energy is so low that I just conk out. Power naps during the day are also a must.

A new pimple popped up on my chin today. Are the toxins escaping? The new breakout could be from the tanning booth yesterday. I got a little sunburned, which is irking me. Tomorrow I vow to take it easy.

Day Seven

Ew, I accidentally put too much maple syrup in the lemonade concoction today. There wasn't enough time to make a new batch. It was really gross, but I think the added syrup gave me a short burst of energy. Cup in hand, I started dancing around the kitchen. Three more days and I will be back to eating real food!

Don't tell my boss, but I spent the first thirty minutes of work staring at the computer. I have a horrible headache today and the computer screen was making my eyes pulsate. The fluorescent lights at work also hurt my eyes. Thank God I didn't really have to speak to anyone all day. It would have been difficult to carry on an intelligent conversation.

My mind is definitely moving more slowly. I think I'll take a sick day tomorrow. I am trying not to be consumed by this cleanse, but my energy was really low at the end of the day. I didn't drink an adequate amount of lemonade because I am getting sick of the taste.

My bowel movements are painful and coming far too frequently. I started drinking less water in an effort to decrease the number of times I have to visit the bathroom. It wouldn't be a problem if I were doing the cleanse at home, but it is embarrassing to use the bathroom a lot at work.

Thankfully my sniffles are completely gone, which is a great comfort. And my sunburn has settled into a golden tan. But my skin smells unusual. Is this from the toxins? The smell might be from the tanning booth and the after-sun lotion I use.

This cleanse needs to end soon because I have become the worst girlfriend ever. I do not have the energy or patience to deal with anyone right now. And my breath smells disgusting. I am continually rinsing with mouthwash.

After I got home from work, I took a long bath and read Scott Fitzgerald's Pat Hobby stories. I started crying, knowing that Fitzgerald died shortly after writing the stories. Cleansing is making me really emotional. That or my hormones are off because I am expecting my period.

I weighed myself twice today and the scale showed two different results. I decided that the lower weight was the accurate one. So according to Mr. Scale I lost seven and a half pounds! My stomach is getting smaller and skinny jeans fit nicely—no more muffin top. I will fall asleep a little easier knowing I'm getting thinner.

Day Eight

Thank goodness it's Friday! I was supposed to go to the office today but I called in sick. Technically I do feel ill. I upped my lemonade intake, and I think that helped get rid of the headache, but I still feel rather weak.

Today I shut all the shades in my house and turned off the lights. I did some stretching exercises in the living room, focusing on my breathing. This gave me motivation to continue the cleanse.

My mother has been calling and insisting that I stop the cleanse. Instead of breaking my commitment, I lied and told her I would stop tomorrow. It is difficult to keep going when people are not completely supportive. Fortunately, my boyfriend has been really great lately. He keeps telling me how pretty my skin looks. I stopped using my face wash and my complexion is radiant.

Our neighbor was grilling outside today, and wafts of barbecue smoke kept drifting into the apartment. At one point, I opened the fridge door and seriously contemplated eating an apple. But I can't stop now. When I set a goal, I have to follow through. I would feel terrible if I broke the cleanse now. And my digestive system feels completely cleaned out. The first few days I was passing gas a lot, but now it's like my intestines have been power-washed. I did, however, consume almost a full package of gum today. Bad move. It intensified the cravings.

My period was supposed to come today but it didn't. I think all this cleansing has thrown my cycle off. Every part of my body is shrinking: belly, breasts, legs. People are starting to notice and give me compliments. I've lost eight pounds so far! Of course this is good news; most women love to lose weight. But I really don't want to focus on the weight loss. I don't want my friends and family to think I am just doing this to starve myself. To me, this is more of a personal challenge, a test of willpower.

Tonight my boyfriend and I packed up the car with blankets and pillows and headed to one of the last remaining drive-in theaters in southern California. The movie was far too long, and I fell asleep toward the end. Still, it was nice to get my mind off the cleanse for a few hours.

Day Nine

I know I'm supposed to ease off the cleanse with fruits and vegetables, but I really want some bread after the final day. Yum, maybe I will have a bagel with cream cheese.

I never realized how many food commercials there are until now. I am probably talking about food too much. My boyfriend's eyes glaze over every time I start talking about my cravings.

Today was really relaxing. I just vegged at home and then went for a short walk to get some fresh air. Again I took the tension off by doing breathing exercises in my quiet living room. I have this little desktop Zen garden with tiny rocks and sand. Arranging the little garden with the miniature rake helped me relax.

Knowing that tomorrow is the last day gave me a boost, but I definitely did not have enough energy today to hit the gym. I can't wait to start exercising again. That is a downside to the cleanse. Also, my breath continues to reek. It is really embarrassing to have to brush my teeth so much.

My monthly friend still did not come today. My digestive system is better, although my stomach is growling uncontrollably. Everything that comes out is very watery.

When my boyfriend and I were cleaning the apartment today, I saw my reflection in the hallway mirror. The pores on my face have shrunk and my skin looks really good. The whole shape of my face has changed. (I seem to lose weight in my face first and my butt last!) All my clothes are loose on me—including my underwear. I swear even my hat fits baggy. But my loving boyfriend assures me that my head is still as big as ever!

My dreams have been really vivid and strange lately. I had this bizarre dream that I was having dinner with the Obamas. I usually don't remember my dreams when I wake up. Now I am sleeping longer and better, minus my usual sleeping pill.

Tomorrow is the last day! It feels like Christmas. I can't wait to wake up.

Day Ten

I made it! I made it! I feel so accomplished. All day I have been laughing and joking. I put on a full face of makeup and curled my hair. Over these ten days my body and mind have completely transformed. In total I lost nine pounds!

My lemonade mixture was really low on the lemons today. I suspect my boyfriend used some more of my prized lemons for his tea. I didn't feel like buying more. To be honest, I didn't drink as much lemonade as I should have, but it doesn't really matter since today is the last day!

I also drank way too much water and had to visit the bathroom nearly every thirty minutes. I have a bad habit of not following instructions. It really does help to follow the guidelines and drink the lemonade first thing in the morning. I've noticed that when I wait until late morning to drink the tea, I'm hungry and irritable for most of the day. Next time I will make more of an effort to drink an adequate amount of lemonade.

Today my boyfriend and I went to his mother's house for a barbecue. He devoured a plateful of ham, potatoes, bread and more. I had to explain the cleanse to his family. I got a few strange looks, but I didn't want them to think I didn't like their food.

Afterward, we went to the supermarket and bought all the appropriate provisions for my first meal—uh, my *healthy* first meal. Okay, I did kind of go overboard, purchasing muffins and frozen lasagna. I am hoping I'll have the self-control to not binge tomorrow. Wish me luck!

I feel like I can accomplish anything now. Yikes, I just realized I didn't do my taxes yet. If I can complete a ten-day cleanse, I can certainly file my taxes. I'll finish them tomorrow, and after that I vow to do something really nice for myself to celebrate.

Joann

Day One

This is my second attempt at the Master Cleanse—I'm determined to complete ten days this time. The first attempt didn't last past Day Eight. My downfall consisted of a brownie and a turkey sandwich, which I gorged on first thing Day Nine rolled around. I was not consumed with hunger for eight days, nor was I feeling sick or weak throughout the entire process. I was, however, suffering from massive, relentless cravings.

I originally decided to perform the detox as a means of mental and physical cleansing. I wasn't happy about gaining weight and eating sweets compulsively at stressful moments. My relationship to food was not balanced: I wasn't giving it the mindful attention it deserved. I believed the cleanse would help cure me of anxiety-ridden eating habits so I could start fresh. After the first attempt failed, I gained fifteen pounds in two months and gorged on more sweets than ever before. The only good thing about this binge was that I discovered a passion for cooking and baking. I started having dinner parties and impressing my friends with meals and desserts, something I'd never experimented with in the past. I baked brownies, cakes, pies, tarts and cookies. I held large dinner parties where I served roast chicken and standing rib roast, baked savory pies and mixed vegetables in a variety of concoctions. I was never not full, and I felt myself getting fatter and fatter. I was eating compulsively, gluttonously, consumed in guilt. After a few months I figured I'd give the Master Cleanse another go, start fresh again—and this time, come off the detox correctly, without gorging. So here I am, on Day One.

Last night I had a final meal of Japanese fried rice with egg and some amazing, gooey sauce. I savored a mixed-fruit tart, a dessert I've been consuming every single day. I went to bed with a cup of senna tea and prayed I would do it right this time. This morning, after I woke up, I drank four cups of the sea-salt flush, using a straw to avoid the nauseating taste overwhelming my taste buds. I followed my usual routine of walking the dog, meditating and yoga stretching. And I waited for something to come out. About half an hour later, out it came—a big, long one. It was a good start to a day, Monday to be exact, and I went to the studio determined and grounded.

I work at an artist's studio where cigarettes are passed around like popcorn and meals are eaten alone in front of a computer. I decided to quit smoking, again, simultaneously with the detox. It felt good to know I wasn't going to fill my pained lungs with smoke. Sitting in front of the computer, checking my e-mail, I felt no urge to reach for that pack, nor did I want to chew gum, or munch on nuts, or what have you. I did feel a bit light-headed and disoriented; perhaps it was nicotine withdrawal, perhaps hunger. My brain is normally restless and anxiety-ridden, at a constant run. Today there was a breeze billowing through the crevices of my mind and I felt free. Perhaps that's all projected, but it felt real.

The first cup of lemonade gave me flashbacks to the first attempt, and I was doubtful for a minute, wondering if I could really do this. Can someone with as little self-control as me achieve something that requires Herculean mind control and discipline? I'm as compulsive as a human being can get. It was a bit ominous: Nine more days. Nine more days. Can I really do this? *Yes, you can. Yes, you can.* I let the evil angel flutter away and repeated my mantras and continued with my day. I lasted through the day drinking six cups of lemonade, craving sweets but not really hungry for food. I came home and drank a couple more servings of lemonade; then, for the first time in months, I went to bed early. I was feeling lethargic and heavy and didn't feel like getting any writing done. Overall, it was a good day.

Day Two

The food obsession has begun. I've spent hours upon hours browsing food blogs, bookmarking hundreds of recipes that sound undoubtedly delicious. The fact that I can't seem to restrain myself from this self-inflicted torture is reflective of my current outlook about this process. I'm depriving my body of food but, more importantly, I feel like I'm depriving my mind and spirit of nourishment.

I woke up feeling pretty chipper and optimistic that it wasn't at all bad; no cramps, no cravings, no pangs of hunger, just following a routine and taking it as lightly as possible. I paid one visit to the bathroom after the heinous-but-tolerable saltwater flush; again, one normal lump. I drank six cups of lemonade throughout the day and was unable to make myself drink any more. I noticed a metallic aftertaste and mucus in my throat, perhaps a result of not smoking combined with the effects of toxins gradually escaping my body. My tongue had a transparent white glow but wasn't as gross as it can get during the fast.

I worked in the studio and succeeded throughout the day in being moderately clear-headed and not minding the nicotine deprivation. I can't say I was productive, though; I was busy finding twenty-eight different chicken recipes using all types of sauces, from jerk chicken to Vietnamese-style honey ginger, to barbecue, to full-roasted herb chicken. It was pure food porn, my substitute for food consumption. By the end of the day my stomach was feeling quite empty, but the guilt I feel from being a gluttonous bloat these last few months has yet to subside.

Friends mocked me when I admitted I was doing the cleanse after vowing I would never put myself through such torture again. The first time, they were there putting up with my whimpers and whines about the beauty of brownies, how each soft, scrumptious, chocolate-chunked bite sends electric currents through your veins, and, oh, how orgasmic it is when bits of coconut are thrown in for good measure, and how unforgettable is the scent, upon walking into the kitchen, of those baking bits from heaven. My friends were sick of it and pitied this pathetic soul. But they also understood, as did I, the benefits of the Master Cleanse—its ability to decompose and neutralize the toxins that have been residing in my body for years. Even more important, it's an opportunity to really start fresh and cleanse the mind of bad habitual thoughts and behaviors. I've tried to talk some sense into myself today, telling myself that browsing food blogs is not the way to cleanse my mind, that this is even worse than binging and that I should really be writing about that art show I've been meaning to review.

But no. My mind won't rest until I've found enough no-knead bread recipes to feed an army. My eyes are bugged, my body ignored, my mind overflowing with dreams of meals. I'm not consumed with guilt; by now I'm used to these self-destructive behaviors that have more or less been my life's path. I've comforted myself to sleep knowing that what I am intending to do with the Master Cleanse is good and healthy, a purification of the mind, body and soul that erases the soot and creates a clean slate.

Day Three

I feel lighter and airier today than I have the last two days. I'm not hungry; I've been eating with my eyes, browsing through TasteSpotting (food-porn site) and hundreds of other blogs, bookmarking millions of recipes.

I haven't had serious urges to eat or smoke. I've been feeling pretty normal, if a bit weak and distracted. I went jogging last night, which felt awesome. I have been going to bed super early, around ten, which I haven't done in years. In the past, I've made it a rule never to crawl into bed before midnight because sleeping is a waste of time and I don't need more than six hours. Well, I've done some catching up the last two days, that's for sure.

For the first two days I didn't have to use the bathroom as frequently as I had expected, which can only mean there's a bunch of shit (sorry!) clogged in there. Today was another matter: I used the bathroom frequently and the stuff was more diluted than what usually comes out. This is good. I think detox is officially starting today, whereas the last two days my body was revving up, preparing to decompose all that nasty stuff in my intestines. This cleanse is the Drano that declogs and cleans up your intestinal pipes and purifies your bloodstream.

I've ignored my stomach rumbles and the light-headed-ness I experienced after getting home from work. I took the pup to the park, but rather than going on our usual walk I sat down on a bench and didn't get up for half an hour. My body was a bit tingly and very tired. The clouds and drizzle seemed to contribute to the lethargy. It's also that very special time of the month (which helps explain why my face is so pale).

A few hours and seven cups of lemonade later I felt better and stronger. Once I got home I was anxious to get some writing done, but instead I ran to my food magazines and stuck a million Post-it notes to awesome recipes. (My roommates warned it wasn't a great idea, but when do I ever pursue good ideas?) Then I decided to be productive with my time and made a list of the reasons I'm doing this cleanse:

1. Rid myself of this compulsive eating habit. Learn to moderate rations and willingly stop eating when my stomach tells me I've had enough. Find peace between mind and body and engage in conscious eating.

2. Lose this heinous belly fat that folds over my jeans and jiggles when I jump. (Shudder.)

3. Start incorporating healthy meals and desserts into my diet. I've just found a few great blogs that will help me do this. No more all-purpose flour and refined sugar; it's time to try oat flour, muscovado sugar, date bars, rolled oats, soba noodles, vegan chocolate cake, homemade granola bars, eggless frit-tatas, chili, tofu, chickpeas, peanut sauce, coconut oil, and vegan cranberry scones. I will never be a full-out vegetarian or vegan. As an avid meat-eating Korean, I would find that very difficult. But I can

limit my intake of beef and poultry to weekly rather than daily.

I always seem to maintain a certain dose of self-destructive behavior. At the same time, I always want to start fresh, wash away the bad, the old, the accumulated junk, to sweep it all away and start clean. That's how I've approached relationships, work, school. It's a process of building up until I just can't handle it any longer—I explode into a tantrum and shout ENOUGH!

The last few months have been great in that I've tried new recipes and ingredients I'd never come across before in my entire life, but I've been eating in such disproportionate quantities that it's damaged my sense of well-being. I've been feeling fat and bloated all the time and can barely fit into my clothes. In the last few weeks, I was just short of not caring—I ate all day, nonstop. It's a cyclical and repetitive complaint at this point, but I'm determined to finish the cleanse and do it right this time. Cross your fingers.

Day Four

I feel just fine today. Just fine. The drastic mood swings from the first day to today might ignite paranoid-schizophrenic suspicions, but at this point I'm just relieved to feel at peace. I went to the bathroom three times from the morning to midafternoon, and each one was far from solid. The exact opposite, actually. I've never been this fascinated by my own excrement, but I think you would be, too, if you realized that thin, wispy chunks were disintegrating from the walls of your intestines.

Today I didn't spend too many hours staring at food pictures, and I actually got some writing done at home. My mind felt calmer, with a steady wave of good thoughts that overpowered the slight craving for a cigarette. I was very proud about not craving a cigarette.

I don't have a husband or children, so I don't have to worry about feeding them or watching them feast without me. I do, however, have friends I've ignored the last few days because all they want to do is go to my favorite crepe house on St. Mark's Place and share a Nutella-banana crepe with me. Or they want to go to that bar with ping-pong tables and drink cheap beer. I've secluded myself in my room, and if I do step out, I make sure to go to events that don't allow eating. I went to watch a documentary at MoMA about the Williamsburg art scene in the '90s. I brought a bottle with three cups' worth of lemonade. The bottle was empty by the time the film was over, and I needed to get home to drink more. I wasn't feeling anxious or hungry, but I definitely wanted to scurry home where I was safe from temptations.

I can mix the lemonade with my eyes closed at this point, and I go on with my day sipping on the drink and taking no mind to the repetition. I have a bit more mucus accumulating in my throat, and that gross metallic after-taste is just nauseating. Today I drank a total of six cups of lemonade. I can't seem to make myself drink any more than that; I just have no interest. I play around with the amount of pepper in my lemonade: I haven't been adding the full eighth of a teaspoon because it's too hot and makes me want to hurl. I've been adding a tiny pinch, and if I feel daring (or guilty for not following directions) I'll add more. I'm aware the portion is important for breaking down the mucus, and it's entertaining to imagine little red critters floating in my intestines kicking some toxin ass, but I can't get myself to add more than a pinch.

No sign of stomach blubber going away. I don't have a scale, so I just eyeball my weight. So far, there has been no change. Pity. Hopefully tomorrow I will shoot out ten pounds into the toilet. Despite being in a chipper and content mood today, I can't wait till this is over.

Day Five

Today was another good-mood day. No irritating mental itches, no barking at the slightly—but harmlessly— disobedient dog, and no intense fog of unproductivity. I have been wasting late-night hours staring at food online. I'm surprised there are no semi-masturbatory simulation-eating toys out there for people who are fasting (this must be my calling).

I did feel an intense sensation of chills today. I was cold the entire day, despite having the heating pad on at max and curling in the fetal position under a thick down blanket. It started yesterday, but it was mild and I gave it no mind. Today it was intense, attacking with full force. My frozen bones were in dire need of a knitted sweater and a mug of steaming hot chocolate. There was only so much ignoring I could do. I went for a brief and easy jog around the park and came home shivering. Mind you, it's winter, but it was mild enough that I would normally come back sweating, with pink, heated cheeks. I definitely didn't feel this chill the first time I tried the cleanse, during the summer. It's disheartening, uncomfortable, and it's distracting me slightly from my writing sessions. This is, luckily, my main physical complaint today.

The mucus in my throat and the metallic taste in my mouth continue; there is a gross layer of white on my tongue. Good news that the detox is working. There is a gnawing emptiness in my stomach that reminds me of eating and makes me want to eat. Today, for the first time since Day One, I felt hungry, but the urge wasn't strong enough to be discouraging. I simply noticed this sensation and moved on. This led me to drink two more cups of lemonade than my norm, for a total of eight cups. I didn't feel myself getting lighter until today, but it finally feels as if the constant bloated feeling that I've lived with for the last few months has passed. Bowel movement was pure waterfall, not a lump or chunk of any kind to be felt or seen. That hurts after a while. I imagine the pepper is what causes the stinging and burning, or perhaps it's actually the toxins leaving my body that are causing the chafe.

At this point, I want to experience the mental and spiritual clarity the book promises on Days Nine and Ten. I fear I might not continue this fast past Day Eight, like the first time. It's getting old. I'm bored and slowly realizing this is not good for my mind or body. The body is smart enough to store fat and food when it receives signals of starvation, and it won't release nutrients till it's fed again. Making my body work this way seems wrong. My body shouldn't be deprived of nutritious food intake, and my mind shouldn't be engorged in this hopeless lust for food. I think this just isn't the right means of cleansing for me. There are hundreds upon hundreds of success stories, shared in websites and forums, of people who happily fast for weeks on end, feeling greater by the day. It simply isn't for me. But let's see what tomorrow brings. I worry too much about the past and the future, and I'm learning to take it one day at a time.

Day Six

These mood swings are killing me. Today is a quintessential bad day. I'm testy and short-tempered; I'm dismissing my friends, my coworkers, my dog, turning into a combination of hermit and angry caveman. I haven't showered in two days out of laziness. I feel existentially dirty. Restlessness and anxiety are my closest friends at the moment, and even my morning yoga stretch wasn't gratifying or releasing. I'm feeling pretty clogged and just getting sick of this cleanse. I simply want to eat. Knowing I'm willfully sacrificing an option to eat feels worse than starving out of poverty. I'm obviously hitting a low point. It's very possible that tomorrow I'll hit euphoria and be blessed with good feelings. But right now I'm in the dumps, discouraged and skeptical, and I want this to be over.

Like yesterday, I was cold all day, shivering uncontrollably from the deepest part of my body. Seems like my body is lacking the nutrients it needs to build heat and energy. The reason might be that I was only able to get myself to drink four cups of lemonade. This lemonade concoction is monotonous and tasteless, and I need change. Now.

Bowel movements were more solid than yesterday, so I'm concluding solidity of excrement is directly linked to my mood. There must be some serious mental toxins being released because I feel potentially hazardous and fragile. I also visited the bathroom a lot today, three times to be exact, each one more diluted than the one before.

I'm surprised I'm not pining for a cigarette or wanting to stuff a burger in my mouth. I do want to eat—I wouldn't label it hunger, but rather a compulsive desire to eat out of stress and boredom. I have a few friends who went on this cleanse, and I thank my lucky stars I haven't experienced their symptoms: headaches, barfing, serious cramps, body aches, sleep deprivation and nightmares. One friend didn't sleep an hour the first two days and was a fogged-up zombie. (I got her into reading food blogs mid-cleanse and she disowned me for it.) The cleanse is hitting me from a different angle, causing my mental toxins to flare up and release themselves with relentless ferocity. Maybe this is worse than having physical side effects, as it has really become a self-destructive process. When I tell people I'm on this cleanse they are initially intrigued, but they eventually pity me. I went to my neighbor's house party and watched with envy as people dipped chips in guacamole and hummus and sipped beer like it was manna raining from the heavens. I was so jealous and antisocial that I had to excuse myself and run out the door.

Today is a discouraging, loathsome day, and it doesn't look like tomorrow is going to shine any brighter. Good thing is, I'm sleeping more than I have in years, going to bed by ten, which was just unheard of before the cleanse. I never allowed myself to go to bed before midnight, but now the more time I can spend being unconscious, the better.

Day Seven

I woke up feeling really cold again and didn't want to get out of bed. It was a difficult morning. I was lightheaded and weak, my joints were sore from God-knows-what and I was generally out of it. I almost forgot the saltwater flush. I didn't snap out of this zombie mode till I had my first lemon juice of the day.

Today I hung out with one of my few friends who is neither dismissive nor sympathetic about the cleanse; he's excited that I'm challenging myself in this unconventional manner. We met at a café (I treated myself to peppermint tea), and he allowed me to indulge in my food obsession. I made a list of things I'm going to cook and bake upon coming off the detox. Some highlights include lemon poppy-seed bread, bananas-Foster bread pudding, granola bars, chocolate-covered coconut macaroons, curry chicken, pork loin with rosemary and garlic, and pesto pasta. Later, we went to the Essex Street Market and browsed through aisles of independent vendors ranging from butchers to fishermen to cheese merchants and bakers. I had a blast picking up stinky cheese and sniffing the hell out of it, and I drooled over the piles of delicious-looking nutty and fruity bread. The caramel-chocolate tart almost made me faint. I made my friend eat a small bread roll while I watched; I made sure to sniff it before it disappeared into his mouth. Why would I torture myself this way? I guess it's better than sitting in front of a computer sulking and complaining. It was fun to experience food in this alternative way, without actually consuming it. But I will admit it was masochistic of me.

I was surprised how much energy I had walking around the city all day with just three cups' worth of lemonade in my bag. I didn't even drink much of it till I got back home—I was preoccupied by all the food I was "eating" with my eyes, nose and ears. But by the end of the day I was very tired and had no energy. I only drank a total of five cups today and couldn't get myself to drink more. I paid a visit to the bathroom twice in the course of the day; both times it was pure brown water.

At least I was in a chipper mood and didn't bark at my friend even once. I tried to get some writing done, but I couldn't keep my eyes open and was too cold to care. I watched a few episodes of *The Office,* snuggling with the pup under the covers, and I soon fell sound asleep. It was an eventful and educational day. I just can't wait till this is over and I can really go shopping—going down all the aisles and picking up every single item that I want.

Day Eight

During the day today I was feeling just fine; it was a good day, in fact. I was energetic, light-hearted, focused and productive. I went to my favorite café for a few hours to get some writing done, took a glance at the croissant and the brioche, waved hello and moved on to the tea list. I treated myself to another peppermint tea. (I'm not sure why the book recommends mint tea and not chamomile, which is also easy on the stomach. I guess mint is more a stimulant and refreshes the taste buds, while chamomile functions more as a soothing downer.) I got a few hours of writing done—in between food-porn browsing and recipe list-making.

I had two watery bowel movements after the flush. It seemed more painful than other days; perhaps my body is just overworked. I went on with my day still feeling sick of the cleanse, performing my duties out of necessity rather than choice. I drank a total of six cups of lemonade.

In the evening I had agreed to help a friend cater a party, clearing empty cups and refilling hors d'oeuvre plates. I walked in determined not to give in and was confident I would do fine. If I had known what was coming I wouldn't have helped out. There were infinite amounts of crackers, olives, cheese, meat, chocolate and wine, and the boisterous crowd made me want to not care. I was laughing and chatting, instinctively grabbing food from plates, only to put it back half a second later.

Then I slipped. As soon as I saw the mound of assorted cheeses and the accompanying meat tray, I salivated and helped myself to a small piece of cheese. This sent a lightning bolt of flavor into my mouth, and suddenly I couldn't control my greedy hands. Next thing I knew I was hovering over the caterer, uncontrollably helping myself to freshly sliced prosciutto and tasting all the cheese blocks. I was unstoppable, a frenzied robot that didn't know right from wrong. I knew I was going to regret this, but at this point all rational thought had left me. Friends at the party tried to stop me, warning that I was going to be writhing in pain very soon, but I was working—they couldn't strap me into a straitjacket and roll me home. So for the duration of four hours, I sporadically indulged in the pile of goodness in front of me between my duties of picking up garbage and pouring wine.

By the time I got home my stomach was bulging out, but still no pain. I drank my senna tea and sank into bed feeling extremely guilty, but also not surprised to have given in that way. I mean, what do you expect? I was surrounded by delicious gourmet foods. How could I possibly not try them? Comforting myself with that reasoning, I went to bed . . . and simply told myself, *it's over.*

After the Cleanse

I didn't have a bowel movement for two days. I was bloated and constipated. On Day Nine I drank orange juice to come off the cleanse, but I couldn't control myself from eating more. I slathered cashew butter on slices of fresh, crunchy, tangy apples and bit into them in ecstasy. I had a full meal by Day Ten, and that evening I let out a big BM. So once again, I've messed up.

I've concluded the Master Cleanse is not the right source of betterment for me. My goal was to reassess my relationship with food, to appreciate its connection to the body, how it nourishes the mind and soul, in hopes that I could learn to eat in moderation, planning properly pro-portioned meals using nutritious ingredients.

From Day Ten until Day Fourteen I didn't stop eating; I was constantly nibbling on something or other. I'm con-vinced this fast was the stupidest thing I've ever done, twice. Why the hell would I deprive my body and my mind of food, knowing how compulsive and obsessive I am, knowing I would only gorge on food shortly after? It didn't make sense, and it still doesn't make sense. It's been two months since the second time I tried the cleanse, and although I've moderated my portions and cut down on sweets, I'm still constantly bloated. I'm convinced there are chunks of cheese and prosciutto from that party lingering in my intestines.

I can certainly appreciate the cleanse's ability to bring clarity to some people, but it's just not for me. I will have to again reassess my relationship to food, with gradual changes in diet and more exercise. I'll have to learn to eat more consciously and mindfully, suppressing the need to constantly stick something in my mouth. No more eating out of stress. No more eating while reading a book or typ-ing away on the computer. No more gorging gluttonously beyond full. I am learning these lessons slowly and taking it day by day to build a healthy relationship with food.

JOURNAL 8

Christy

Day One

This is Day One of my second Master Cleanse. My first ten-day cleanse was almost four years ago, and let me tell you, it was *not* the most incredible experience of my life. In fact, I consider it to be one of the hardest things I've ever done. I'm realizing now that perhaps that was due to the fact that I didn't do the Master Cleanse correctly. Yes, I made the lemonade every day and I drank it, but there were key elements I either didn't understand or simply ignored.

During my previous attempt at the Master Cleanse, I tried to guzzle the internal saltwater bath. The idea was that the faster I went, the less painful the whole experience would be. Boy, was I wrong! Guzzling made me sick. Unable to stomach the entire quart of water, I gave up on it. Thus my cleanse began without the significant cleansing benefits of the saltwater flush.

Today I approached the saltwater bath with far less urgency, and it worked. I spent close to twenty minutes of my morning nursing a full quart of warm saltwater. I still got a little queasy, but I kept thinking of it as a broth or soup of some kind, and somehow I got through every last drop.

I have felt pretty energetic all day. During my last attempt I constantly felt sluggish and tired, even on Day One. But I don't think I drank enough of the lemonade on my first try. I didn't like the taste of it, so I drank more water than anything else. This time around, I've made a conscious decision to not only drink the lemonade when I feel hungry, but to drink it regularly enough that I don't even begin feeling hungry.

For the past week, I've been mentally preparing myself for this cleanse, something I did not do my first time around. The past few days I've reminded myself of what is to come and thought long and hard on all the reasons it's important to me. I also made it a point to savor each and every bite of those last few meals. Because of this mental preparation, my body hasn't felt all that shocked by the new meal plan.

It is also extremely helpful that my dear husband has decided to change his diet for the next ten days to encourage me. He isn't doing a full Master Cleanse, but he is altering his meals enough to make me feel as if we are embarking on this challenge together. A little support goes a long way.

Day Two

I decided to start the day off by drinking the saltwater again. My resource materials say it's all right to do it every day if necessary. Again it took me over ten minutes to drink the entire quart. The first half went down pretty well. The last half was terrible.

About thirty minutes later, I felt a huge rumble in my belly. That saltwater goes straight through you; it's amazing. I can't explain how great it feels to know you've flushed out your entire digestive system. The only drawback I can think of is that the flush takes a long time to complete. I need at least ten minutes to drink the salty beverage, then it's at least another thirty minutes before it starts to take effect. You need another hour or so to make sure that the flush is complete. No one wants to be in the middle of the grocery store only to realize they have one final run to the bathroom in them. I think that's one of the reasons they recommend you begin the cleanse on a weekend.

Okay. The lemonade. Well, let's just come out with it! The lemonade is not great. In fact, at times it is downright awful. The only time it tastes incredibly good is right after the saltwater. After I drink my third or fourth glass of the lemonade, my stomach starts to ache. I think it's the cayenne pepper. I read tonight that it's okay to build up to the tenth-of-a-teaspoon amount, and I think I'll start that tomorrow. I'd rather pull back on the cayenne and build back up than be queasy every time I drink the lemonade.

I haven't felt overpowering hunger pains yet. I do miss cooking and sitting down to dinner with my husband. That's something we've always enjoyed together, so it seems strange to drink my meals from a cup. But I just remind myself that this isn't forever, and the benefits will far exceed the sacrifice of a mere ten days.

Today I took my dog on a two-hour walk, something I never imagined I would be doing on a liquid-only diet such as this. It was wonderful. I had incredible energy the entire time, but for some reason when I got home I felt exhausted. The first thing I did was mix up another lemonade, and that helped a little, but since then my energy has been low. Perhaps I shouldn't have gone so long without the lemonade, and maybe the two-hour walk could have been cut in half.

As I look to the future, the next eight days seem daunting. A part of me dreads what is to come, believing I can't go that long on nothing more than lemons and maple syrup. But I've done it before. And I'm still here, aren't I? So I'm trying not to think about the next eight days too much. One day at a time. That's what will get me through.

Day Three

Today I didn't do the saltwater flush. In fact, I think I'm done with them. I don't want to overdo it and flush vital bacteria from my system. I also pulled back on the cayenne pepper—just enough that the lemonade feels better going down. I plan to build up to a tenth of a teaspoon in the next few days.

Another element of this cleanse that I didn't follow correctly the first time is the instruction to make the lemonade fresh every time. On my first cleanse, I just wanted the entire process to be as easy as possible, so every morning I would mix together two liters of lemonade and take it with me to work. You think the lemonade is bad now, try it after it's been sitting at room temperature all day. Yuck.

This time around, I'm preparing each glass separately and drinking it within ten minutes. It's made all the difference in the world. While the lemonade still isn't the most delicious beverage I've ever had, at least it's fresh. When I'm on the move, I just mix the lemon juice with the maple syrup and bring that with me, keeping it as cool as possible. Then, right before mealtime, I add the water and cayenne. It's not as difficult as it sounds; it just requires a little preparation.

I realized today that my mouth tastes different. It's incredibly acidic. As a result, I'm brushing my teeth more often, but that taste doesn't really go away. It's slightly bitter; I'm not sure how else to describe it. I've read that during the cleanse, as your body is ridding itself of toxins, these little things can happen.

Day Three feels very difficult. I remember from last time that Days One through Three can be the biggest challenge as your body adjusts to the new routine. The best strategy for me is to remain active. I've kept my mind on my work, trying to be as productive as possible. I find that if I put the focus on my to-do list, time flies, and before I know it, I've forgotten that a pile of lemons is waiting for me at home.

This brings me to the many benefits one can gain from this cleanse. What better time to examine those nasty little habits or unfulfilled intentions? That's how I've been trying to fill my days. I'm taking a hard look at the choices I consistently make and how I generally use my time. How have I been eating, loving, growing, learning and giving in the past few years? In what ways do I continue to disappoint myself and/or others? And I'm suddenly realizing how much work I have to do. It's a little overwhelming. In fact, it makes Day Three feel like a walk in the park.

Day Four

Today feels much easier. Now that I'm over that third-day hump, I think my body is starting to adjust. I've felt a huge surge of energy all day. Of all the fasts I have tried, this one feels the best because you are still consuming solid calories that will push you right through the day.

I have to say, though, that I don't think this is the kind of thing one should do frequently. A lot of thought and preparation should go into each cleanse or fast. To do it on a whim, or just to lose weight, doesn't seem like the best motivation. Let's face it, anyone can lose weight on this cleanse. You're downing nothing but liquids for ten days! But what happens when the fast is over? What next?

If you use the Master Cleanse only to lose weight, without seriously analyzing bad habits, the underlying problem will rear its ugly head again in time. If there is no change of heart or mind during this process, once you move back to solid foods you will gain every single pound back. Don't bank on a magical change overnight. There's no quick fix when it comes to eating and living well. It takes great dedication and an understanding of how your body responds to food and exercise. This cleanse can be the beginning of that remarkable effort.

For me personally, the point of this cleanse isn't to lose weight but to evaluate all aspects of my life as I detoxify. Four years ago, I did use this diet as a means to lose weight. I lost ten pounds, but it didn't last because I didn't take this time to question or explore my mentality when it came to food.

My life has changed significantly since that time, but I remember how difficult that was for me and I don't want anyone else to make the same mistake. It's beyond frustrating to work so diligently for a result that slips right through your fingertips.

Day Five

One of the most difficult aspects of this cleanse, I am remembering, is the fact that life continues around you. My husband eats breakfast, lunch and dinner. Though his meals have been modified, he's still taking part in normal everyday routines that I am not.

Your couple friends are still inviting you over for dinner and your girlfriends want to try that new restaurant downtown. Your coworker still offers you a doughnut every morning and your neighbor still brings over that banana bread she just baked. Even someone's simple gesture of offering you a stick of gum or a piece of candy can suddenly feel earth-shaking.

There's just this constant fork in the road directly in front of you. Do I continue going down the path that I have chosen? Do I push forward and complete these ten days without cheating? Or do I forget it all and just live my life the way I always have?

Stretching and challenging oneself is never the easy road, but it is the most satisfying one. Because what happens when you give up? You go to that restaurant, enjoy a great meal, then come home and long for a change in your life—the very change you just gave up for a few hours with friends (a pleasure, by the way, that you can enjoy anytime after these ten days are over!).

It is difficult. That's for certain. Because I don't want to be "that girl." You know, the one who can't enjoy pizza with everyone because she's, *gasp*, on a cleanse. There's this constant assessment of who you can share that information with. Most people I've told have been incredibly supportive, but a few have gone into a tizzy. They argue that the cleanse isn't legitimate, or they question your self-esteem.

It can feel as if you are leading a secret life. You share the information with some friends, and to others you become "Missing In Action" for ten days. I'm not quite sure how to juggle it most of the time.

Day Six

I got called in for jury duty. And today I woke up really late! In my haste to pull all my paperwork together, get directions and take the dog out, I completely forgot to bring my mixture for the lemonade! I didn't remember until I got to the courthouse around 8 a.m. I'm very much a breakfast person these days, and I completely walked out the door with nothing at all in my belly. Misery. That's what this morning was.

As I sat there filling out my forms, waiting for my name to be called, I spotted a vending machine in the corner. Only a dollar or two could make my stomach stop hurting and remind me how to spell my name. But I couldn't do it. Not only did I not want to sabotage the cleanse, but absolutely nothing in that machine looked appetizing. Wow. That's a big change. Normally, most everything in a machine like this would be calling my name. No temptation today. Just misery. And I actually longed, *longed* for that blasted lemonade. I couldn't believe it!

Luckily, I was released for the day at 11:30 a.m. I almost skipped down those courthouse steps! "Here I come, lemons! Almost there, maple syrup!" my heart cried. And when I got home, I immediately mixed up a nice, cool glass. Ah, liquid lunch.

Well, I learned a lesson. Tomorrow I'm getting up extra early to make sure this doesn't happen again, because chances are I won't be let out early next time. Jury duty. Always putting that big kink in your plans.

Day Seven

Three more days! I cannot believe how quickly the time has gone by. I mean, there have been moments I could have sworn time was standing still, but now it feels like I blinked and it's already Day Seven. I feel great, and I'm confident the next three days will fly by too if I just give myself over to the process.

My husband continues to be supportive. His diet has wavered a little, but for the most part, I see him making sacrifices to stand in solidarity with me. I feel very blessed to have someone in my life who is personally invested in what I'm doing.

I've been able to build up to the tenth of a teaspoon of cayenne pepper, but it still feels like way too much. It just makes me queasy. Tonight I'm going to read through my resource materials to figure out exactly how little of the cayenne I can get away with.

My mouth still tastes incredibly acidic. It makes me worry for my teeth and gums. I've been brushing my teeth like a madwoman to keep the lemon juice from eating away at them. When I think back on this cleanse, I just know I'll suddenly get a strange taste of cayenne pepper and toothpaste in my mouth!

I cooked a meal this evening for my husband. He was in a hurry so I made his dinner while he got ready to leave. I don't think I could have done it on Day Three, but today, having just consumed a nice, tall lemonade, I was happy to throw together a healthy little concoction for the man I'm crazy about. Avoiding the kitchen had been making me sad, as I truly love to cook. What would have been very difficult a few days ago ended up being a very relaxing exercise for me today.

Which brings me back to this idea of evaluating one's life while on the cleanse. I wonder what would happen if, during this cleanse, we all focused on loving and serving other people. How much more enjoyable it would be! I've spent the better part of the last seven days thinking about myself. What this means to *me*, how *I* feel, and how *I'm* hungry or not hungry. What if that energy was turned outward, putting the focus on those around me? What more could be learned? Uh . . . lemonade for thought, my friends. Lemonade for thought.

Day Eight

Some people claim that on the Master Cleanse they've been able to take up extreme workout regimens due to the amount of extra energy they have. As great as I feel, I don't think I'm strong enough to go on a run or lift weights. I feel good enough to take long walks and to continue going about my daily tasks, but anything more than that would be too much for me. I don't want to push too hard and strain my body. An intense workout can burn several hundred calories, and I'm not pulling in that many calories to begin with.

I'm remaining active throughout the day, taking my dog for a walk or to the dog park, running errands, working and writing. I did carry some heavy groceries home (a ten-minute walk) the other day. And I pumped each bag up and down like a free weight, working out my biceps. But that was enough to make me feel like a rag doll by the time I got home.

I have lost a little weight, but I'm trying not to dwell on it. I'm pretty much where I want to be in that regard, so gaining those pounds back carefully in a few days is definitely a goal. I think it's helpful to set a desired (yet healthy and realistic) weight and stick with it, no matter what the world may tell you. Women are constantly bombarded with unrealistic images and expectations of what our bodies should look like. It's difficult not to buy into it. Yes, we should all strive to be healthy. But skinny and healthy are not always the same thing.

I want to feel confident in my clothes and I'd prefer that my weight not fluctuate much either way. Constantly losing and gaining back weight is harder on your body than simply maintaining. Women should encourage each other to eat well, live well and love ourselves for who we are.

Day Nine

I read recently that some people on the Master Cleanse experience strange bodily odors from the release of toxins. I haven't noticed any change in the way my body smells. I have, however, been sweating a lot more than usual. It might be due to the fact that I'm drinking more water. I've been remarkably active these past nine days, plus it's spring and the weather is getting warmer.

I have yet to find a conclusive answer to my cayenne problem, but I've reduced the amount again. I'm a little tired of making these lemonades. The fact that they have to be made fresh every time is a bit of a burden. A few times I've almost skipped a needed lemonade meal because I was frustrated by all the squeezing and measuring and mixing. It would be so much easier if I had a juicer. Not only would it take half the effort, but I'd be able to get so much more out of each lemon.

Judging by the way I feel right now, it'll be a while after the cleanse before I go back to eating anything that contains lemon juice, maple syrup or cayenne pepper. The lack of variety is one of the hardest things about this process. It's made me realize how spoiled I've been. I mean, before I began this fast, breakfast, lunch and dinner rarely looked the same. I hardly ever even ate leftovers! Now every single liquid meal is identical, right down to the tablespoon.

I don't really feel hungry today, but I am craving variety. I just want something else in my mouth besides what I've been tasting the past nine days. Maybe that's another reason I'm brushing my teeth so often. That cool mint flavor is a refreshing change.

I can't believe tomorrow is Day Ten. What once felt light-years away is suddenly one night's sleep from now. I'm so excited, I may not even be able to sleep.

Day Ten

What can I say? It's Day Ten, and I can barely believe it. It almost feels like Christmas—this exciting day that's been hovering in the distance that I thought would never arrive. Now it's here and I'm simply giddy.

I am looking forward to returning to a normal meal schedule. I've read that you shouldn't just move right back to your usual diet. That is definitely one part of the cleanse that I ignored four years ago. Once the ten days were over, I went right back to my regular foods. This time around, I'm really going to make an effort to slowly adjust back to solids. Since I've come this far, I might as well go that extra mile.

These past ten days have been a great time to stop and think. Sometimes it's nice to slow life down a little. Don't get me wrong; it hasn't been easy. But it was much more difficult four years ago when I didn't follow the instructions. There's a reason you are instructed to drink at least three liters of lemonade a day, to drink it fresh and to drink it often.

Today I plan to spend a quiet day contemplating exactly what this process has meant to me. One of the things I've been thinking about is the fact that we live in a culture where the act of denying oneself is rarely embraced. If we want something, we waste no time in getting it. The concepts of "want" and "need" can start to seem like the same thing, but it is important to be aware of the distinction between the two. Sometimes the very thing we long for is, in actuality, harmful to us.

JOURNAL 9

Genevieve

Day One

I woke up early this morning to discover that the laxative tea does indeed work. Cramps woke me and I was forced to get up and go to the bathroom. The cramps weren't as bad as I expected, and after I went to the bathroom three times (the stool wasn't exactly normal, but it wasn't diarrhea, either) I crawled back in bed and fell fast asleep. I woke up again at 9:30 a.m. and was ready to start my day.

I was surprisingly awake and ready to have my first cup of the lemonade, but first things first: the saline rinse. It was a little hard to swallow a whole quart of saltwater, but I did it. I imagined it was a giant dirty martini, my drink of choice, and that actually helped. The saline rinse affected me the way it was supposed to: thirty to forty-five minutes later it was all out of my system.

I then prepared my first lemonade. I had been wondering about the taste of the lemonade, and when I tried my first sip I was pleasantly surprised. I love citrus fruits. The only thing I didn't like about the lemonade was the pure maple syrup. I've never been a huge fan of maple syrup, and I could definitely taste it in the mixture.

I tried to watch TV but I couldn't sit still and focus on the show. I suddenly had all this energy. I felt jittery, like I had downed a couple cups of strong coffee. This feeling lasted all day, so instead of relaxing I had to find ways to occupy myself. Usually I sleep in, and some days I don't have much energy, but today I ran all my errands and still had time to spare before my boyfriend came home from work.

My food cravings today were bizarre. When I drove by fast-food restaurants I felt tempted, even though I haven't eaten fast food—or wanted to—in six months. After I finished my errands I watched a movie, and I craved everything they were eating in the movie. The characters drank coffee, which I love, and ate cake and croissants. Usually I never think about food during the day unless I'm figuring out what I want for lunch or what to cook for dinner. Today I thought about food all day long, and at the end of the day I was mentally drained. I felt as though I had taken food for granted and now I couldn't eat any.

I'm trying to be positive about this experience because I truly believe that you control your own success. I decided to do this cleanse because I have had stomach problems for years. So far, my body seems to be reacting just fine. I did notice that I was biting my fingernails today, and I usually only do that when I am anxious or nervous. I also noticed that I'm not as introspective. I am always lost in my head, but today I was all about the moment, planning what to do with my time. It was really refreshing. I hope this way of thinking continues as I go on with the cleanse. I know if I can make it through the first couple of days I will soar through the rest.

Day Two

This morning I woke up early again and had to go to the bathroom. It wasn't as bad as yesterday, but still I was in there for about fifteen minutes. I went back to bed and woke up again around 9:30. This morning was different. I didn't have any energy. I got up and made the laxative tea and then drank my first lemonade. I got back in bed and watched TV. At least I could focus on the shows. I ended up getting really absorbed in a *CSI* marathon and that occupied my mind for several hours.

It wasn't till about one o'clock in the afternoon that I started thinking about food. But once I started, I couldn't stop. For the rest of the day I struggled with whether I could finish this cleanse. At the lowest point in the day, I forced myself to take a shower. In the shower I decided I wasn't going to quit. I don't want to give up on anything that I start. My sister called when I was out of the shower and I told her how I really wanted to cheat. She was outraged that I was considering giving up so easily. We talked for a while and she helped me realize that I wasn't a quitter and this cleanse would make me a healthier and stronger person. My sister suggested that instead of looking at the whole thing as ten long days I should look at it as one day at a time.

I headed to the bathroom at least seven or eight times during the day. One thing that happened to me today was I experienced the mucus I had read about. It was very strange to see big globs of mucus coming out of me, but it was also sort of interesting.

I was really negative today, and I hate being negative. I noticed that I was more impatient than usual. I got frustrated with my sister because there was a lot of background noise when we were talking on the phone. When my boyfriend got home from work, he was talking to someone on his cell phone and I almost lost it. I needed him to distract me so that I wouldn't think about food! But I didn't yell at anyone, so at least I can still control myself.

Day Three

I woke up at 2:30, 4:30 and 7:30 a.m. to go to the bathroom because of the laxative tea I drank last night. I also had stomach pain throughout the night. This morning I was extremely tired, but I got up like clockwork at 9:30. As I mentioned earlier, I usually sleep in, but I haven't been able to on this cleanse. When I woke up, my stomach felt completely empty, as though I had thrown up all night.

Even though I had a rough night, I was excited about starting the day. I did the saline rinse and it worked just the way it had before. Yellow and brown water flushed out of me. As the day progressed, I had a good amount of energy and could focus; it was a complete 180 from yesterday. I worked out today and felt fine. I plan to work out even longer tomorrow and see how I do. I now believe I have gotten over the hump.

I enjoyed drinking the lemonade today. I increased the amount of lemonade I'm drinking because I felt really hungry last night. I drank ten cups today instead of seven like yesterday, and that seemed to help.

I didn't crave food as much as I had on the previous days of the cleanse. I actually watched a cooking show and it didn't bother me at all—I even got some ideas for healthy meals I can cook when I'm done with this cleanse. I was disgusted by a show that featured ground beef and described how it is made. I was also disgusted by a fast-food commercial that showed a lot of different kinds of fried food. I hope it's a healthy sign that I am no longer craving junk food.

I weighed myself today and I have already lost two pounds. My stomach looks amazingly flat. I haven't noticed any other physical changes, but I think in the next couple of days I will see more.

It's strange, but I even think I was nicer to my boyfriend today. I thought about how much I appreciate him. When he got home from work we had a great time just hanging out together. He has been very supportive of me during this cleanse and it's helpful to have him in my corner.

My emotions have been up and down since I started the cleanse two days ago. I was a mess yesterday and today I was happy and optimistic again. I can only hope that the rest of the cleanse makes me feel as good as I did today.

Day Four

I'm starting to notice that every night I drink the laxative tea it works a little faster than the night before. Last night I woke up about two hours after I drank the laxative tea. My night was pretty rough; I got up at least four times to use the bathroom.

This morning, just as every other morning on the cleanse, I woke up at 9:30 a.m. I drank the saline rinse, and about five minutes later it started coming out of me. The saline rinse is working faster on me, too. I had stomach cramps that persisted until the rinse was completely through. I haven't seen any big globs of mucus today, only small pieces of mucus and bile.

I sniffed my armpits before I got in the shower this morning and they smelled very strange. They didn't smell like BO or deodorant, and it took me a couple minutes to figure out that they smelled like hair-removal cream. I have used a depilatory cream maybe three times in my entire life, and never on my armpits. The more I thought about it, though, the more it made sense. Those products contain lots of chemicals and during this cleanse my body is releasing trapped toxins.

I lost another pound, for a total of three pounds so far. I haven't seen much of a change in my body, but my boyfriend said I looked really skinny. He is actually worried about me. I tried to explain to him that I'm drinking my meals, and that lots of people have done this cleanse, but he didn't get it. Then I explained to him that I am cleaning out my body in an attempt to alleviate my chronic stomachaches. He understood that I'm not doing this to lose weight but to make myself healthy again.

My energy level is up again, just like yesterday. I'm feeling good mentally and physically. I was sort of hungry during dinnertime, and I started thinking about Mexican food. I started craving chips and salsa, guacamole, and a bean and cheese burrito. I made myself a glass of the lemonade and I was fine.

My stomach feels as though it has shrunk. It won't stop growling, but I'm not sure I would be able to eat very much if I could eat. I started a list of foods that I want to eat when I'm done with this cleanse. The list includes mostly healthy foods, like artichokes, strawberries, broccoli, shrimp and spinach.

Day Five

Today was an extremely hard day. It all started with waking up at 4 a.m. because of the laxative tea. I had bad stomach pains and I felt like I had to go to the bathroom, but nothing would come out. It took three trips to the bathroom for something to finally come out, and even then it wasn't much.

While I was in the bathroom, I had a breakdown. I felt so nauseous and sick that I started questioning all the reasons I started this cleanse. I wasn't feeling healthy or happy at all. I finally went back to bed. I was so drained from waking up in the middle of the night for four days straight that I managed to sleep until 10:30 a.m.

I lay in bed for a while until I had the strength to get up and prepare my saline rinse. I had no energy, and I longed for the days of waking up and eating breakfast. As usual, the saline rinse went right through me. I was surprised that I still had a lot of stool and bile in me.

I also got mad at my boyfriend today. He asked if I wanted to go to a barbecue at his boss's house tomorrow and I told him I didn't want to go because I'm still on my cleanse. He said that he had already committed us to the barbecue, and that he had told his boss (and the boss's wife) that I wasn't eating. This pissed me off because I didn't want anyone besides my boyfriend and my sister to know I was doing this cleanse. I didn't want to have to explain the cleanse to everybody. At their last barbecue, the boss's wife asked my boyfriend if I ever ate because I didn't eat her chili (I don't eat meat). Now she will probably think I'm crazy or anorexic. This bothered me for most of the day, and I finally called my boyfriend later in the day and told him I couldn't go to the barbecue. I didn't want to explain the cleanse or watch a bunch of people eat right in front of me. In the end, he understood, but I was still annoyed by the whole thing.

This has been the hardest day since Day Two. I'm not craving food; I'm just feeling weak and frustrated by everything. I decided not to drink the laxative tea tonight because I really need a full night of sleep. I don't think I'm breaking the rules: the book says you can stop the laxative if it makes you feel sick.

I weighed myself and I haven't lost any weight since yesterday. I also haven't seen any other physical changes. My breath smells like the lemonade, and my body smells normal to me. I'm glad I don't stink. I'm not sure I could handle it today.

Day Six

Today I woke up at 9:30 a.m. again and was pleasantly surprised that I had energy and a good attitude. I slept through the night without waking up a single time. I really needed that, and I think it put me in a better state of mind.

I drank my saline rinse and, like clockwork, it flushed right through me. It only took about a half hour for the entire rinse to pass through me. I didn't see any bile today—just yellow liquid.

I recommend staying out of restaurants and grocery stores when on this cleanse. Today I sat with my boyfriend at a restaurant and watched him eat a burger and fries. I thought I was strong enough, but all I could think about the whole time was how much I wanted to order something. I imagined reaching over and grabbing just one french fry off my boyfriend's plate. But I've come too far to give in now. I stayed strong and drank my glass of water instead.

For the rest of the day, I was craving all kinds of junk food. I watched a show that profiled a doughnut shop in Oregon; the doughnuts looked so delicious. The weird thing is I don't even eat doughnuts. I can't remember the last time I had one.

I have noticed some physical changes today. My nails are stronger. I've been growing them out, and whenever I grow my nails out, one of them always ends up breaking. But they are stronger this time—none of them have broken yet. I also noticed that I am having a breakout on my back. I guess it's just the toxins coming out of my body. When I weighed myself I had lost another pound, for a total of four pounds. However, my weight seems to fluctuate depending on the time of day.

Even though I had a hard time at lunch, the rest of my day was fine. I just drank more lemonade to distract myself from cravings. The thought that kept me going was "only a few more days and I'm done!" I remember Day Two, when I almost quit. I feel like I'm becoming a stronger person on this cleanse.

Day Seven

Last night I drank my laxative tea earlier than usual, hoping it would make me go before I fell asleep. Instead I was up all night with stomach cramps. I wanted to go to sleep, but I was afraid I would not wake up with enough time to get to the bathroom. I ran to the bathroom three times and nothing came out but gas. I finally had some results at 4 a.m., but after that I still felt like I had to go for the rest of the night. It was horrible. It was probably the worst night I've had since the second night. Fortunately, I only have a few more nights after this.

Today was a really hard day. My boyfriend and I got into a huge fight. All I could think about was whether we were going to make it through this. Part of our fight was about the fact that he thought I was starving myself. The whole time I've been doing this cleanse he has been flip-flopping on his support.

It was hard to be cleansing and have emotional turmoil at the same time. Today I felt I needed to eat something because I was emotionally and physically exhausted. I tried to stay busy during the day to keep my mind off the cleanse. My sister is moving soon, so I went over to her apartment and helped her pack up stuff and take clothes to Goodwill. At one point, she told me she had some chocolate-chip-cookie-dough ice cream in the fridge. I reminded her I was still doing the cleanse and she felt bad. A while after that, I asked her if we could eat the ice cream, but she wouldn't let me. She reminded me how far I have come and that I only have a few days left. Instead of giving up, I drank one of my lemonades.

I weighed myself and I lost another pound. I haven't noticed any other physical changes besides the fact that I feel exhausted. I was so tired by 10 p.m. that when I lay down I fell asleep instantly.

Day Eight

Today was much easier than yesterday. My boyfriend and I made up so I could finally focus my mind on this cleanse. I was able to relax, regroup and realize that I only have two days left. I finally got a good night's sleep last night, but I was still sort of tired today. My legs were sore and I felt like I needed to relax.

I noticed that my armpits smelled like hair remover again. It's weird, but if there are bad chemicals in my body, I'm glad I am getting rid of them. I weighed myself again and I have lost yet another pound. I have lost a total of six pounds, but I'm not sure where the weight is coming from—I haven't noticed any big changes in the way my body looks.

At about 2 p.m., I started having cramps. They weren't stomach cramps; they felt more like menstrual cramps. I'm sure I'm going to get my period tomorrow. It got so bad at one point that I had to take a Tylenol. I'm not sure if that's against the rules of the cleanse, but I had to—I was in pain. I hope my period doesn't bring on any weird food cravings. Usually when I'm on my period I eat more and I crave sweets like chocolate and brownies.

I've noticed that my boyfriend has been eating fast food. We never eat fast food because I usually cook a healthy meal with a protein and a vegetable. It is interesting that I'm getting healthier on this cleanse and he is eating worse. He had McDonald's tonight for dinner and it didn't bother me, but I did sort of watch him eat his burger without him noticing. I almost feel like I should cook for him even though I can't eat, but that would just be ridiculous.

I had an epiphany today that the human brain is an amazing instrument. If you put your mind to something, you can achieve it. Now that I have seen this firsthand, I am going to use it in every aspect of my life. I truly believe I am going to be a more successful person when I am through with this cleanse.

Even though I was tired during the day today, I stayed up till 11:30 p.m. because I just couldn't fall asleep.

Day Nine

I woke up with more painful menstrual cramps. I slept in till 10:30 a.m., then I got up and drank my saline rinse, and just like every other day the rinse flushed through me almost immediately.

The cramps made me pretty sluggish. I stayed in bed for a couple more hours after completely passing my saline rinse. I didn't have much energy, but I was excited that I'm almost done with this cleanse. I did start to get more energy as the day went on.

I ended up watching a cooking show, but instead of craving the food, I just wanted to cook it. I decided I would make my boyfriend a home-cooked meal. I wrote down the ingredients for a red-wine-marinated flank steak and a sweet onion salad. I needed to go to the grocery store anyway to buy lemons for my lemonade, so I decided to pick up the ingredients for the meal, too. In my checkout line, they were offering samples of fresh, sliced strawberries. The checker asked me if I would like to try some. Although I desperately wanted to, I declined. I have never been in a checkout line that had fresh strawberries before, and the one time it happened I couldn't enjoy them!

As I cooked my boyfriend dinner, I wasn't tempted by the food I was handling. It felt a little strange to serve him food I hadn't tasted, but he said the steak was the best he had ever had.

I did crave sweets today, which I kind of expected since I got my period. I kept seeing this Baskin-Robbins commercial for a Snickers ice-cream shake. The combination of chocolate and ice cream looked amazing—I was lusting after that drink all day.

Looking in the mirror today, I noticed some physical changes that I must have overlooked before. Some of my bones are showing that weren't before. My ribs are more pronounced when you look at my chest. It doesn't look bad, but I don't think I should lose any more weight or I might start to look anorexic.

I drank my laxative tea tonight for the last time. I was so excited to be done with it. I know I will probably have to get up and go to the bathroom tonight, but it's fine with me because it's the last night.

Day Ten

Wow. I can't believe I made it to the final day. Last night I couldn't get to sleep at first because all I could think about was everything I wanted to do today. I wrote a to-do list and couldn't wait to start it.

I had a great night's sleep. Even though I drank the laxative tea, I was able to sleep the whole night through. I didn't go to the bathroom until I woke up this morning, and I only had to go once. I got up around 10:30 a.m. and drank my last saline rinse, and it flushed right out.

I ended up finishing all the tasks on my to-do list with time to spare. I noticed my energy level was remarkably high. I did a few things that I usually procrastinate about, like replying to e-mails and submitting my writing samples.

I cooked my boyfriend dinner again tonight and I wasn't bothered by it at all. I didn't crave any particular food, but I did start to get hungry at 7:30 p.m. so I drank my last lemonade. Making that last lemonade felt so freeing.

I have to admit that I thought about the food I am going to eat when this cleanse is over. I am going to follow the food plan that was outlined for after the cleanse. Tomorrow I start by drinking fresh-squeezed orange juice, and the next day I will incorporate vegetables and soup.

I am excited about Easter brunch on Sunday. It will be my third day off the cleanse, and I'll make healthy food. I don't want to become unhealthy again after this cleanse. I plan on eating organic and cooking my own healthy meals at home. I don't want to gain back all the weight that I lost, so I plan on working out to maintain my weight and to get more toned.

I am astounded that it is Day Ten. If someone had told me on Day Two that I was going to finish this cleanse, I wouldn't have believed them. My mind is ready to take on bigger challenges now, and I feel extremely optimistic about the future. I feel that this cleanse has made me healthier, stronger and even happier with my life.

Day Eleven

Today was my first day off the cleanse. It was weird waking up this morning and not drinking the saline rinse or lemonade. I felt almost attached to the lemonade and didn't want to stop drinking it.

This morning I felt great and had tons of energy. The first thing I did when I got up was work out. Then I made myself fresh-squeezed orange juice for breakfast. For lunch I ate two oranges. I got hungry again later, so I ate a third orange at 2 p.m.

I think the lemonade drink gave me more energy than the orange juice I ingested today. I was extremely hungry and I craved food all day long. I kept thinking about eating a fresh roll of sourdough bread, but I want to stay healthy, so I decided to drink vegetable broth for dinner. I wasn't supposed to have the broth today, but I only had a little, and it was low-sodium and organic.

This morning I talked to my sister and she congratulated me. I felt so proud of myself. This was one of the toughest things I've done in my life.

Day Twelve

Today is my second day off the cleanse. I was hungry all day. I had two oranges for breakfast, then I went and got my car serviced. When I got back around midafternoon, I was starving for lunch. I made myself vegetable soup with zucchini and yellow squash. It tasted good, but I was still hungry. I started craving a fruit smoothie after lunch and I was starving again by dinnertime. I resisted the urge to have that smoothie, and for dinner I had more vegetable soup. I thought I wouldn't be able to eat much because my stomach has shrunk from the cleanse, but I was wrong.

It might sound weird, but I actually miss being on the cleanse. It got to be a routine and now I almost feel guilty for eating food instead of drinking the lemonade. I think it is going to take awhile to get used to eating again.

JOURNAL 10

Flash

Day One

After I woke up and took a bath, I got dressed up
(slacks, button-down, tie, blazer and nice shoes) to go
shopping for supplies. Already had plenty of grade B maple
syrup; needed lemons, cayenne pepper, sea salt and some
good water to get things started. Got all my supplies then
came home and did my first saline flush. YUCK! I had
woken up early so I decided to take a siesta. Got up again
around noon and made a batch of Master Cleanse mix.

I wanted to get some steam time in to help with the
detox process, so I went to the gym and did a few rounds
through the sauna and steam room. Once I was back
home, I got into some scrapping (mixed-media collage).
I've been collecting a lot of scrapping materials and was
ready to fully dive into it. This fast is, after all, about getting rid of the excess. I also sent out a few texts to my mom
and to my friend J, who said she would be my "fast
buddy" and check in on me every so often.

After finishing the first batch of Master Cleanse mix, I
tried another round of the saline flush. So far I hadn't

really noticed any effect from the first saline flush (perhaps because I went to sleep shortly after drinking it); however, this time I felt it right away. As for the results, everything was pretty solid and normal. A while later I decided on another bath (I haven't taken two baths in one day for years!).

I have done up to a three-day fast before, so I didn't really have a hard time with food cravings today. But that's not to say I didn't notice food (Taco Bell, Starbucks and a pizza place).

My fast is taking place in a basically empty house, so I don't think I'll be interacting with a whole lot of people. I wanted to make sure I had plenty of space and time alone to do inner work during the fast. I intend on doing a lot of yoga, meditation, dreaming and healing during the next nine days. I'm very interested to see how my life changes in such a short but potent time.

Day Two

So I'm kind of craving food today. Mainly foods I've had recently that I really enjoyed: pizza, nachos and baked goods. It surprises me how much power thought has. Throughout the day, I'd be thinking about how hungry I was, and then I'd shift to thinking about my fast and committing to it, and all of a sudden my hunger would just go away.

When fasting, my awareness increases dramatically. One of the biggest themes that shows up in my thinking is abundance versus lack. When I feel like I *lack* food, I start to get hungry, low-energy, apathetic; whereas when I focus on the abundance in my life, I feel full, energetic and ready to take on anything.

A great example of this type of energy shift happened today. I needed to get some household supplies so I went to the store. On the way there, the weather was really rainy and cloudy. Walking by all the food in the store, I was feeling that lack in my life. But after I bought what I needed and got back in the car to drive home, the clouds instantly broke and the sunshine was brilliant.

Part of the reason I planned this fast is that I realized there would be a lot of value in slowing down my pace and taking time to just sit, breathe, and do nothing. At the same time, I didn't want to get in a thought rut and not get anything done. So in my "down time," one of my goals is to get more in touch with my creative energy.

Also, while I'm not eating, I've been giving more thought to mindful eating and having a much healthier diet. I'd like to start eating more yogurt because it hast healthy bacteria and a lot of protein, and it's good for digestion. I've never been vegan for a long period, but I'd like to do that as well to see how it affects me. I've thought about it before and the thing I would miss most would be cheese. It's one of the main sources of my protein right now (that and peanut butter!). Ideally I'd like to find a yogurt-like product that isn't dairy or soy, because too much soy leaves me feeling sluggish. I'm really into smoothies, and I want to learn more about really good, high-quality ingredients for them.

I added Emergen-C to the saline flush—much more palatable. At this point: liquid in, liquid out. It surprised me a bit, but my skin is already starting to look healthier and I'm noticing an increase in the speed of my physical healing. I have a small cut on my finger that is healing more quickly than normal.

I noticed when I feel like I have a purpose in doing something, it's much easier. This is such a great opportunity to clear old energy and get new habit patterns going.

Day Three

Woke up from dreams of cheese! Also, in my dream, someone told me that I stink. I kinda do. That's good, though; it means I'm getting toxins out of my system. I've been getting plenty of sleep lately to help facilitate healing. Again I mixed Emergen-C with saline for my flush, and I think I'll keep doing that for the rest of the cleanse.

I went for a walk after getting up and I really tapped into this feeling of being solar-powered. I could feel the sun pouring its energy into me, almost like I was a battery being charged. I also feel like my senses are heightened. The colors of the sky, grass and flowers were awe-inspiring. It was like the saturation knob was dialed WAY up.

I'm beginning to feel more fluid. Walking feels like dancing. And the consistency of my skin seems to be changing—it has a natural shine or glow to it. I'm also getting more and more into my art. I've got a sketchbook that I've been drawing in.

When I give myself permission to heal and to let go, things tend to flow a lot better. I keep thinking about slowing down, not doing anything and just being in the moment. I've definitely been working on my Zen practices, like "watching the world go by."

Above all, I feel really joyful and happy just to be alive. Last year, I wrecked my Astro van. Not gonna get into that story, but I definitely feel that this cleanse is part of a process of rebirth.

Day Four

Dreamt of cheese balls last night! Two nights in a row. Guess I'm craving cheese! "Cheddar" is also slang for money, and I want that, too. Funds are running low, but I know things will turn around. I feel like I'm doing the inner work right now so that external forces will align.

I have been looking for a job. I move around a lot and am nomadic, which I feel often holds me back when it comes to being employed. I need a job that I can move around with. After talking to my mom today, I started to focus more on *thriving* rather than surviving.

On a walk earlier, I felt blissful just breathing. The cold air in my lungs reminded me of home and of being in the mountains. It was great to have the experience of being *fed* by air.

My car was starting to have some problems today, so I went and got the part I needed and fixed it. I'm not that big into cars, so it was very empowering to get in there and do the repairs myself. Perhaps I was inspired by the healing work I am doing on myself during this cleanse.

Thinking about food a lot more today. This is the longest I've ever gone without eating. I want Mexican food. As much as I feel like eating, I feel like cooking even more. I really want to barbecue tofu. Make some really yummy pita pockets, or some homemade pasta.

Sometimes I feel asocial. It's not that I don't like people; it's just that I really enjoy being alone and having my own personal space. Getting to know myself during this fast has been a great experience. This whole process is very cathartic, and I feel that I'm gaining a much stronger foundation by achieving a state of balance.

Day Five

I went to the library this morning and, while walking home, I felt the presence of this emotional wave rising and falling within me. I feel like it will soon swell to a point where I start crying, which I haven't done for a long time.

I was reading today that during the Master Cleanse your body can potentially release stuff that's been accumulating for decades. Here on Day Five, I thought there were no more solids left in my body, and I figured I wouldn't be eliminating anything solid from my system. But today a bunch of gunk that I think had been stored in my system for a long time finally found its way loose. Very happy about that!

I am having some major food cravings today: doughnuts, English muffins with butter and honey, bagels with cream cheese, spinach with peanut sauce, peanut butter, and orange and cranberry juice. After this fast is over, I want to make a HUGE pot of soup. I've got all the fixings for it, and I've been waiting for the right time.

Today I found out there is a Vipassana silent meditation sit on Saturday (Day Seven!) and I think I'm going to attend. I did a longer ten-day sit the winter before last. It was a powerful experience, and it helped me gain a feeling of focus and determination that I'm now finding crucial during this fast.

My dreams have been really clear lately—one of the many benefits from fasting. Another odd effect is that I feel like I can hear electronics! I think this is just from my senses being heightened. Speaking of electronics, today I've been thinking that humans are basically virtual machines. Our minds and bodies are organic computer systems that can be programmed, and right now I am in the midst of defragging and reformatting my "bio-computer."

Day Six

Last night, after writing in this journal about a bunch of foods I wanted, I had dreams of eating. This morning I called and got the info I needed for the Vipassana sit. Then I started the day off doing some housework for the lady I'm staying with. I felt sluggish and tired. I think doing some stretching and maybe going for a run would be a good way to get my blood flowing.

I'm looking for another housing situation, as this one is only temporary while the house is for sale. I'd like to get into a communal housing environment. I need to get a job first, though, so I can procure some funds. I had an interview today for a job in social-media marketing.

After my interview, I went back to the place where I crashed my van. I hadn't been there since I crashed last year. There were still pieces of my van on the side of the highway. Crashing my van has been haunting me, so it was good to go back there and face it. While driving home, I got to thinking about the importance of enjoying life and appreciating everything. I started to think about eating and how when I break this fast and begin eating again it will be slower and much more mindful. More chewing. More tasting. More savoring. I also started thinking about putting more positive energy into the food while preparing it.

When I got home I sat in the bath, gazing at the flame of the candle that was burning by the tub. All of my senses are so alive. I feel *at one*. I was feeling hunger in my stomach and then I started thinking that I *am* nourished. All of a sudden my stomach rumbled, shifted and I felt very full. Amazing! It's very inspiring to me how capable we are when we decide that we will accomplish what we set out to accomplish. I feel like nothing can stop me. More than that, I feel like everything is actually here to help me. I'm so grateful for this journey that I'm on.

Day Seven

I had a late-night talk with a friend that was emotionally draining. Although I feel very nourished, I still don't feel like I have a whole lot of excess energy to pour into others. I wanted to get up and go to a yoga class this morning but I was just too tired. I thought about sleeping in even more and missing the Vipassana sit, but I finally dragged myself out of bed and got going.

I put less salt in my saline flush today because Mom was worried about me (she works at a doctor's office and is always keeping a close eye on my health). I also doubled the amount of Master Cleanse mix I'm drinking. I was kind of surprised that I didn't have a bowel movement at all today.

I did the half-day Vipassana sit. It was great to refresh my memories of the teachings that were a pivotal turning point in my life the first time I sat. It's nice to just sit and observe what *is*—good and bad—and know that it will pass. I had a moment where I was starting to get hungry and bored, but I decided that I was going to just sit it out. As soon as I made that decision, my stomach did the rumbling thing (almost like a little kid getting over a temper tantrum) and then the ending meditation started. It's amazing: As soon as you "allow" something, it passes much more easily.

After the sit, I met up with a friend at Café Gratitude, a raw food restaurant. He was eating a macro bowl. I'm excited about getting back to eating, but at this point I feel like I could fast indefinitely. I think I hit this yogic threshold. I don't even feel like I need the Master Cleanse mix, or water, or anything. All of a sudden these things that had seemed to be my huge sustainers no longer seem to be important. I'm plugged in and that is enough.

After we left the restaurant, my friend and I sat outside and played guitar/freestyled. A guy passing by stopped and listened for a while. After we parted ways, I headed to the steam room again. I wanted to get in one more good steam before my trial membership at the gym expired.

Got home to great news: I got the job! I decided a bath was in order. More candle-gazing.

Day Eight

Woke up from a flying dream! It's the first one I've had that I can consciously recall. Before I started flying in the dream, I saw the man who took me to my first Vipassana sit. He's also the one who introduced me to the Master Cleanse. Coincidence? I think not.

After waking up, I went out to buy more lemons and water. It was fun to walk through the store and smell all the lovely smells. That was enough. I don't need to eat the food—smelling it brings its own satisfaction.

On the way home, I saw a yard sale and stopped to check it out. I ended up buying a little two-person dome tent and some craft supplies. Then I went home and set up the tent! I'm not big into nature or anything, but I felt so connected with my yang energy and with being a man. I felt rugged, manly and independent. All from setting up a tent in the backyard!

Once I had set up the tent and put my bedding in it, I sat and did some meditation. After meditating for a bit, I made some Master Cleanse mix with the supplies I had gotten. I was surprised to realize that it was late in the afternoon; I'd only had water and a bit of herbal tea and I wasn't hungry or anything. My body is doing really well running on less. It's becoming more efficient with the resources it does have.

I don't smell bad anymore. That's a great sign. A lot of toxins must have passed out of my system by now. I was really hoping the white stuff on my tongue would have cleared up, but it hasn't. Oh well. I was also hoping my eyes would be clear and white. There's still redness, but there is more clarity in my eyes.

I think I'd like to make a software application that lets you keep your stats for Master Cleansing—a simple tracking tool for the various aspects of the fast (weight, intake, output, emotions, thoughts, dreams, etc.) so that it'd be really easy for people to record what they are going through and look back on it later to see how much progress they made.

Day Nine

Slept in my tent in the backyard last night. It was really windy and I kept thinking that maybe someone was outside the tent. I woke up around 2:30 a.m. and was really cold, so I went inside and took a nice hot shower. I ended up falling asleep on the couch. Early in the morning, I went back outside and got a few more hours of sleep (there was some daylight by then, so it wasn't as cold).

After waking up, I started to craft some business cards. Each one is unique; I wanted to do it that way as a symbolic reminder to myself that each contact I make is also unique. While crafting, I felt really joyful. At one point, a huge smile burst across my face as I thought to myself, "I love my life!"

My afternoon flush was really, really dark. Blackish. I'm getting some dark toxins out of my system. I'm happy about that.

I'm really excited about my new job. It's exactly the job I was hoping to get. I feel like doing this fast allowed me to get all my "blockage" out of the way, clearing a path for my dreams and goals. My friend in Berkeley also said he has some extra work that I could do. So basically I went from no job to one and a half jobs. Nice!

I need to find some really good sources of protein. So far I've got: beans, nuts, cheese, tofu and spirulina. I'm really excited about the spirulina. I used to drink it all the time with orange juice, but I never realized how much protein it has in it. I also need to make sure I'm getting all my vitamins and, based on my talks with a nutritionist I know, some good probiotics. I can't express how excited I am about tomorrow. I plan on ending my fast at the Hare Krishna temple (they have the best food!) once it's dark out.

Day Ten

Happy 22nd birthday to me!

This morning's saline flush was to be my last. The saline flush has been my least favorite part of this fast. I put the saltwater on the stovetop to warm up (so the salt would dissolve a bit). Then I got on the computer and became so engrossed in what I was doing that I forgot all about it! By the time I remembered and came rushing out, the water had mostly boiled off. No flush, I guess. Happy birthday to me!

A while later, I got ready to go up to Berkeley to celebrate my birthday. Before I left the house, I went through all my stuff and picked out some items I wasn't

THE MASTER CLEANSE EXPERIENCE

really using that much and put it all together as my birthday present to People's Park (there is a place in the park where people leave free stuff). Then, Master Cleanse mix in hand, I set out to the park. After dropping off my bag, I went and checked out a couple of nearby bookstores. After I had read all that I could read, I headed over to my best friend's house.

She was surprised to find out that I had been fasting for ten days (but not *that* surprised because I had been hanging out with her a lot when I did my three-day fast). We chatted for a while and then I was off to the temple to eat! When I got there the place was packed. It was a festival day. It felt so nice to be in a spiritually charged environment; especially after ten days of fasting and on my birthday.

I contemplated just taking food home and waiting till the next day to eat. I sat down for a while, then a lady came up to me and asked where my plate was. I told her I didn't have one yet and she quickly took me to get a plate. She started to serve me food and I asked her not to give me very much, as I had been fasting. The look she gave me made me bust up laughing! She asked me why I had been fasting and told me that eating food as pure as *prasadam* (a meal, like today's feast, that has first been offered to the gods) was the best thing you could do to get rid of all negativity. The people at the temple are so cheerful and positive. I'm glad I went there. After I was done eating, I went outside to where this kid I know was sitting with a woman I hadn't met. We all started talking, and it was so nice to be hanging out with people and just enjoying myself. I hadn't done a whole lot of socializing while fasting.

Later, when I got home, I took a quick shower and sat down to reflect on the past ten days. I'm happy about all that has happened during this time, and I know there is so much potency in this experience that it will take me a while—weeks? months? years?—to digest it all.

Samantha

Before the Cleanse

It's the night before I begin the Master Cleanse. I am nervous and excited at the same time. I know I should really be easing into the fast, but I'm craving sushi, and since I will be unable to indulge in such an extravagant meal for quite some time, tonight I'm taking myself out for a nice sushi dinner. It will be my temporary farewell to food. I am also rationalizing spending the money on this meal, as I will be saving plenty by not eating for ten days.

I've decided to do the Master Cleanse for many different reasons. First, I am hoping to rid my body of toxins. Aside from my alcohol intake, I consider myself a very healthy person; I am active and eat a well-balanced diet. However, there appears to be so much processed junk in food that is impossible to avoid unless you cook all your meals at home. It is very disappointing that even organic foods contain numerous fillers.

I have heard that the Master Cleanse can be a great way to treat several ailments. I have ulcerative colitis and I do not like the medication I am using to treat it. Currently,

I am taking two hydrocortisone Cortenemas twice a day. This process requires that I lie on my side for a minimum of thirty minutes. My only alternative would be to take pills every day. I am hoping that fasting will give my colon a break, relieving my current flare-up. Lastly, I am also secretly hoping I will lose some weight. I realize anything lost will most likely be gained back shortly after the fast is broken, but I can't help but want to drop a few pounds.

Day One

I started the day with the saltwater flush: one quart of lukewarm water with two teaspoons of salt. I must say it is nothing short of disgusting. If the water wasn't warm, I might be able to gulp it down more easily. I managed to get the entire quart down in about three minutes by plugging my nose while I swallowed. The flush nearly made me puke. I did in fact gag—twice.

I am pet-sitting my brother's dog. This morning the dog needed to go out, but I was hesitant to leave on his morning walk because I was worried I would need to use the toilet. Good thing I waited as I needed to go almost immediately—ten minutes after I drank the solution.

Throughout the day I noticed my mouth getting dry. I wasn't that surprised; this is common for me if I go too long without a meal. I took little sips of water here and there, and that helped somewhat.

The Master Cleanse book says I should be having a BM several times a day. I have not had a BM today, though I generally don't use the toilet every day. I'm a bit irregular and often constipated. I usually go every few days. I'm concerned about not using the bathroom each day I'm on the Master Cleanse, as I know the detox will be helping me to release toxins and waste, and it's important for this to exit my body. I decided I should drink the laxative tea tonight and do the flush each morning. I wasn't planning on doing this, but upon consideration it seems like a good idea.

In terms of activity, today I took it somewhat easy at the gym. I did twenty minutes on the exercise bike and twenty minutes of stretching. I also spent plenty of time walking around the city. I weighed in at 149 pounds.

I went to Whole Foods to stock up on organic lemons, organic grade B maple syrup and spring water. I was a little shocked by the bill. This diet isn't exactly cheap. I did choose to buy the high-end brand of maple syrup rather than the generic store brand, and that cost quite a bit more.

About the lemonade—tastes good, actually. I'm not quite using two tablespoons of maple syrup, as it seems a bit too sweet. I'm using more than an eighth of a teaspoon of cayenne pepper, as I love anything spicy. I only drank four cups today. I make it fresh each time, as it gives me something to do. I normally spend a lot of time cooking, so on this cleanse I feel as though I'm suddenly given a lot of extra free time.

Overall, I don't think my first day was too bad.

Day Two

Today I popped up at about 5 a.m. with incredible stomach pain from the laxative tea I drank last night. The pain was absolutely horrible, but as soon as I went to the bathroom, it subsided.

I started my morning with the saltwater flush. I still gagged, but at least this time I knew what to expect. It took a little longer to kick in, but it did eventually go right through me.

At the gym I did the same workout as yesterday, but I also went swimming. I made some extra lemonade in the morning so that I could carry it around with me as I ran errands. I am normally quite hungry after the gym, so I knew I would need something to keep me going.

I noticed that my stomach felt very empty when I got up in the morning, and all throughout the day I was a little weak. Each time I drank the lemonade, I felt better. It really did manage to satisfy my food craving. It's hard to believe a liquid diet can manage to keep you going all throughout the day, but somehow it does the trick.

Today is much harder than yesterday. Food smells are driving me mad. It was today, on Day Two, that I realized this diet will be quite difficult. I already started thinking of the first meal I want to have when the fast is broken. My senses feel heightened and my nose has transformed into that of a hunter in the woods seeking out my next kill. I also just feel a little strange. If I could make up a word, it would be "wizzy"—not quite dizzy, but not quite normal, either. My eyesight is weird, and I feel sort of dazed. I also have a lot of mucus and my ears are clogged.

Today, I drank five cups of tea and about two cups of water. Before going to bed I drank the laxative tea again, but this time I didn't brew my cup nearly as strong. Hopefully I won't wake up with stomach pains.

Day Three

The laxative tea kicked in around 5 a.m. again, but this time the stomach pains were far more bearable. I probably could have gone back to sleep and dealt with it later, but I decided to get up. I began the day as usual with the saltwater flush.

Before I began the Master Cleanse, I was having a colitis flare-up, which usually consists of gas, diarrhea and anal mucus/discharge with blood. My symptoms are still there, but it is only Day Three so there's hope.

The mucus from my chest is getting worse, and now I appear to have green phlegm. (This could be from a previous cold.) I have a constant runny nose and a very dry mouth. Water does not seem to help my dry mouth—somehow I think I will have it throughout the entire fast.

Today I momentarily forgot I was on the cleanse and, upon leaving the kitchen, I almost reached into a bag of nuts for a little snack. It wasn't because I was starving but more out of habit. I usually grab a handful of something or other when I leave the kitchen, whether it's nuts, carob chips or tortilla chips. I'm glad I didn't cheat, but I came very close.

I did my usual gym routine, but today I upped my workout to thirty minutes on the bike, along with some lap swimming. I went into the steam room as well. I weighed in at 146 pounds. I drank about three glasses of water and six glasses of the lemonade.

Before going to bed, I drank another glass of the laxative tea and I remembered to brew it fairly weak.

Day Four

In the morning the laxative tea worked like clockwork. It is becoming my alarm clock. It's a little earlier than I'd prefer to wake up, but the tea is doing what is expected so I can't complain. This time was a little bit different, as I had to go again after I got up at 8:30 a.m. I didn't think it would be necessary to do the saltwater flush after using the bathroom twice in the morning, but I did it anyway. I decided I will do the laxative tea every night for the entire cleanse, followed by a saltwater flush in the morning. I think structure and routine are important on this cleanse.·

This morning I was not hungry. My stomach feels fine, but I force myself to drink the lemonade anyway. I prefer to sip on it even when I'm not particularly hungry or in the mood. I'm a person who would normally eat all day long, so I worry that if I go for too long without the tea, I will get insatiably hungry and the tea will no longer be able to satisfy me. Today I drank about six cups of the tea and two regular cups of water.

The symptoms of my colitis are finally beginning to fade. I did not see any blood today. Oh, how wonderful it would be if the cleanse would clear up colitis flare-ups! I could finally say goodbye to those horrible hydrocortisone enemas.

I'm noticing that I am weak. I am not tired, just weak. Each day when I'm walking up the hill on the way back from the gym, my legs feel weak. It seems like the hills have gotten steeper, and I'm finding myself wanting to take a taxi back home. This is not my norm. I am usually a very active walker.

Tonight I survived my first dinner out. My friend was having a birthday party at a Mexican restaurant. I would have skipped the dinner, but it was a birthday so I offered to go as the designated driver. I wanted to enjoy a beer or margarita with my friends, but I kept reminding myself that it was only for one more week so I could sacrifice one dinner out. Honestly, it wasn't too bad watching everyone eat and drink, but at one point I found myself wanting to suck the salt off the tortilla chips, or chew on something and spit it out. I refrained, of course. I treated myself to some fresh mint tea during dinner. Having a different taste in my mouth was a treat, but it didn't quite make up for the lack of food coming in my direction.

The oddest part of the meal was the reaction from everyone when they heard what I was doing. Everyone kept apologizing for eating in front of me and avoiding eye contact. I thought this was rather strange. After all, I was doing the cleanse by choice so they didn't need to feel bad.

I have noticed that my social life has suffered due to the cleanse. I can't go out and meet anyone for food or drinks (unless it's mint tea). Usually, most of my socializing is done at bars or restaurants. It's amazing how much our culture is centered on food and consumption. I guess it is something you don't realize until these rituals are taken away and you are able to step back and process what is really going on around you.

Day Five

Today the laxative tea woke me up at 3:45 a.m. No sign of blood from my colitis. I'm beginning to wonder, though, if the symptoms will return immediately after I start eating again. I'm trying to be hopeful.

I messed up the saltwater flush and didn't put enough salt in it. I was able to drink it a little more easily than I normally can, and after about an hour of waiting I realized I'd only measured about half the amount of salt I needed to make it effective. I decided to redo the saltwater flush. It eventually worked, but I began to wonder if drinking all this salt was bad for me.

The smell of food is still driving me mad. It's so bad that even the smell of dog food is wonderful to me now.

My tongue seems to be turning whiter. I'm a little disappointed, as I have heard that my tongue needs to turn pink in order for me to be fully cleansed. I'm feeling as though I have a "fuzzy tongue" or "cotton mouth." I've been drinking tons of water, but it isn't helping that much.

I've heard there are ways to cheat on the Master Cleanse without causing any damage, so today I decided I'd research it online. Unfortunately, the book I found online is not free so I decided against buying it. At this point I am going a little crazy, so I spent about three hours doing a search trying to find cheating tips online for free. I did manage to discover a few, but in the end I decided not to cheat. Someone said that vegetable broth is okay, and apparently there is an African root of some sort that can help you deal with hunger. I was hoping to discover that I might eat some sort of solid food because the chewing and food texture are what I miss most. I am finding that my only enjoyment when it comes to texture is chewing on the lemon pulp and rind when I get to the bottom of my cup of tea.

Day Six

Went to the bathroom around 7 a.m. It was nice to be able to sleep in. Maybe my body is getting used to the tea and it is less effective or takes a little bit longer.

I noticed after doing the saltwater flush that the liquid coming out of my body is still brown. I am wondering when it will clear entirely, as I have not eaten for six days. Later this afternoon I had a somewhat-formed bowel movement, but it was only a small amount. Hard to believe my body has not processed everything I had eaten six days ago.

The dry mouth is becoming unbearable. I am brushing my teeth over and over just to take away the horrible taste that has taken over my poor mouth and tongue.

I can't believe I'm on Day Six. By tomorrow it will be a week, but then there's still quite a bit of time left. I keep trying to think in terms of one day at a time, but it is getting more difficult. The cleanse isn't pleasant. It's not that hard, but it's not pleasant, either.

After doing my normal routine at the gym, I weighed in at 144 pounds. This feels great to me. I prefer to weigh around 140 pounds, but I usually weigh closer to 150 pounds. I'm 5'8", so I think I am about average.

I am finding that I'm no longer hungry. I drink the tea more out of routine and to keep my energy level up. I miss the idea of food, but I'm not actually hungry. It's strange to feel satisfied, considering I have not eaten for nearly a week.

Day Seven

Today I am noticeably weak. My vision is entirely back to normal, unlike those first few days. I actually feel quite good, aside from the feeling of weakness. The fuzzy coating on my tongue is beginning to come and go, which is better than having it all day long. I suspect that I am not drinking enough water, and maybe this is why my tongue and mouth are so dry. I start forcing myself to drink water regularly, whether I am thirsty or not.

When I woke up this morning around 7 a.m. to use the bathroom, I had a very odd movement. It was mucus-filled, but different from the way my colitis normally is. I wish someone could analyze my bowel movements for me. Too bad there isn't some sort of Master Cleanse professional out there to answer all my questions.

I am now starting to get paranoid about the lack of protein in my diet. I realize the book assures that we get enough protein naturally, but I somehow don't find this sufficient. Otherwise, why bother eating meat at all? I am recovering from a leg surgery and trying to build the muscle in my leg, so the lack of protein is beginning to scare me. I realize I probably should have asked my doctor about this before starting the cleanse. I also have a prosthetic device implanted in my leg, and I started worrying that the toxins being released might cause some sort of infection. I guess it's a little late to be worrying about it now.

I am noticing the weight difference and, I have to say, I love it. My skinny clothes are beginning to fit better. I can use the tighter notch on my belt. I'm trying to figure out how I can keep the weight off after the cleanse. Perhaps I'm just losing water weight, in which case it will surely come back quite fast.

Day Eight

Had my usual morning consisting of a bowel movement, saltwater flush, then another movement. I find myself wanting to end the cleanse today, but my tongue isn't quite clear yet.

I realize it's supposed to be a ten-day fast, but I am going out of town this weekend and competing in an Iron Chef cook-off and I would like to be able to taste my food and that of the other contestants. I want to ease off the cleanse properly rather than immediately drinking alcohol and eating solid food, and I'm not sure I'll have time for a gradual transition if I fast for the full ten days. I feel certain that if I don't break the fast properly, I will not only get sick, but I will be disappointed in myself for ruining everything after such a good week.

I am beginning to wonder if my tongue has always been white and I just never noticed. I have started to go around and ask people to stick out their tongues so I can assess whether their tongue is whiter than mine. Seems silly, but the friends who are healthy have pink tongues, and the heavy coffee and alcohol drinkers all have white tongues. Interesting.

In the end, I decide to stay on the cleanse and not cut it short.

Day Nine

Today I am very alert. One more day! I am feeling surprisingly good today. Something about knowing the end is near, or that there's a light at the end of the tunnel, is making me very happy.

My tongue is, unfortunately, still white. I am trying to increase my water intake and brush my tongue regularly, hoping to rid myself of the white-tongue syndrome, but it isn't working. I have resolved to stop the cleanse on Day Ten regardless of whether my tongue is clear or not.

My energy level is increasing. I'm back to a regular workout routine. I am doing as much as an hour of cardio, stretching and weights, along with swimming, followed by twenty minutes in the steam room. I am now noticing an indescribable energy. I feel lighter and healthier. It feels like a natural high. I am very proud of myself for getting this far.

I had two bowel movements, both of which were mostly liquid. When I weighed myself at the gym, I was 142 pounds. I love it. I am probably drinking about seven to eight cups of lemonade a day now, and I find I am using more maple syrup. Licking the spoon I use to measure the maple syrup is also very satisfying. I am quite addicted to the syrup now. I guess it really is my lifeline. Without it, I think this cleanse would be impossible.

Day Ten

Last day of the cleanse, and I can finally be done with
that awful saltwater flush! At this stage, the flush doesn't
bother me as much as the bowel movement does. I didn't
manage to pass anything significant this entire time. Some
people say they clear gallstones, but that wasn't the case
with me.

I am proud to say I have no more trace of my colitis
flare-up. This is absolutely terrific, but I do wonder if it
will come back immediately once I begin to eat again. I am
hoping it won't, but I just don't know.

My mouth is no longer dry, but it isn't pink yet, either.
I can accept this, but I am disappointed. If it weren't for
the food competition this weekend, I would continue with
the cleanse.

I plan to do a sped-up version of what the book
recommends for coming off the cleanse. I will do the
orange juice in the morning, then the broth that afternoon,
followed by the broth and vegetable chunks in the evening.
It's not exactly the right way to break the cleanse, but I
don't think I will get sick if I eat and drink slowly and in
small portions.

I'm apprehensive about breaking the fast. My body
feels exceptionally good. I wonder how I would feel if I
continued on the diet. Would I feel even better? Have more
energy? I've decided I will try the cleanse again at some
point, but next time I will try it for two weeks instead of
ten days.

I now believe the cleanse is mind over matter. It's not
so hard as it is annoying. I could have cheated at any point,
but it's about willpower.

After the Cleanse

For breakfast the first day, I drank fresh-squeezed organic orange juice. I diluted it with water and drank it ever so slowly. For lunch I drank it again, but I also had a homemade vegetable broth with very little salt. It was the most delicious broth I've ever had in my life. For dinner, I ate the vegetables with the broth and it was heavenly. It also felt healthy to break the fast with such goodness.

It took me a long time before I had my first bowel movement after the fast. This scared me a bit. I almost wanted to drink the laxative tea, but I decided to hold off. My colitis stayed away for about a week, but it did manage to come back shortly thereafter. By the end of my cleanse I got down to 141 pounds. I managed to keep off the weight for nearly a month.

On the whole, I am very happy I did the cleanse and I will definitely do it again. I am hoping it will be easier next time around, now that I know what to expect.

Holly

Let me start by giving you a little background. I'm 35 years old and I have a relatively active and healthy lifestyle. I've been happily married for eleven years now and my husband and I have a 3½-year-old son. We have always wanted two children, but we've had a difficult time conceiving. We were together eight years before we had our son and have been trying for another child since he was 6 months old. This is where the Master Cleanse comes into play.

What I am about to write in this journal is very graphic and even embarrassing. I am going to tell you everything that happened to my body on the Master Cleanse. To do so, I have to put aside all vanity and ego. I just have to hope that in the future I am not known as the girl with all the goop!

I first heard about the Master Cleanse after I got injured training for the Honolulu Marathon and my doctor sent me to a physical therapist. During my frequent therapy sessions I mentioned to my physical therapist, Chris, that I was having trouble conceiving another child. I mentioned that I was uncomfortable with my doctor's suggestion of fertility drugs. Chris told me about *The Complete Master Cleanse*. He explained that he does a cleanse about every three months and feels great. He went on to tell me about women who have had difficulty getting pregnant and who have conceived after doing the cleanse. I thought to myself, this guy must be crazy if he thinks this special drink can help me get pregnant . . . but what if he isn't crazy? Well, that night I ran to the bookstore and purchased the book. If there was even a slight possibility that the Master Cleanse would help me conceive, you better believe I was going to give it a shot.

I read the book in one day. I came to the conclusion that I might have a prolapsed transverse colon. Tom Woloshyn writes that when a woman's colon falls, it rests on her uterus, ovaries and bladder, causing a host of problems. It seemed to make perfect sense: I am a woman who has had problems with constipation for the last ten years. I sometimes get jealous of my husband's magical ability to have a BM every day! The constipation most likely means that my body is failing to cleanse the colon regularly.

I was also a little freaked out about the possibility of having parasites in my body. I almost felt scared to move forward with the cleanse in case I did find a parasite. It almost seemed as if some things were better left not known!

My next step after reading the book was to purchase everything on the shopping list. Let me tell you, it is not easy to find sixty to eighty organic lemons at the health food store in Hawaii (some items are very limited on the islands). Fortunately, a friend of mine had an organic lemon tree in his backyard and he was able to provide me with as much fruit as I needed. The next item was maple syrup. I was stunned to realize that I would potentially go through two quarts of maple syrup. I have never really cared for maple syrup so I was not looking forward to drinking two quarts in ten days. I soon discovered that when you purchase good syrup it tastes very different from the popular brands. I did spend about $120 on grade B maple syrup. (Again, it is much more expensive in Hawaii.) I then purchased good drinking water and have continued to do so even after the cleanse. I already had the cayenne pepper, so the next item was the herbal laxative. I had no idea what kind to buy. I asked someone at the health food store and they were very helpful. I got the impression that people who work at health food stores love talking about bowel movements. I mean, they were incredibly helpful and excited to hear about me doing the cleanse. This particular person had done the cleanse before so she went on and on about what happened during her cleanse. You will find that when you finish the cleanse, you somehow are less likely to be embarrassed talking about your bowel movements. In a way, you are proud of what you were able to eliminate from your body.

My last order of business before I started my cleanse was to get my family on board and explain everything I was getting ready to do. I highlighted and read excerpts from the book to my husband, John. I asked him to be in charge of preparing dinners for the next ten days for himself and for my son, Maximus. He agreed. He was actually very excited for me. One thing about my husband: I sometimes think that he has more faith in me than I do. It is helpful and encouraging to hear from him that I can do anything I put my mind to.

This cleanse is not easy, but if you are determined, you can do it with great ease. I believe you have to be ready for the cleanse, and I would compare it to being ready to stop smoking.

Day One

My first day happened to be Halloween. Boy, what a day to choose for your first day. I am sure my husband was pleased, knowing that he would be the only one raiding our son's Halloween candy this year. I considered starting the cleanse on the next day, but I came to the conclusion that then I would just have more toxins to try and rid from my body.

I did not deviate from the book; I followed the directions as if my life depended on it. The night before the cleanse I took my herbal laxative, and in the morning I prepared for the first of many internal saltwater baths. Okay, let's stop here and chat about the internal saltwater bath. Well, it doesn't sound that bad. It sounds as if it would be a piece of cake, right? Wrong. The internal saltwater bath is hard to get down. Believe me, though, once you do it, you will never regret it. I think the laxative companies should be worried about this little secret getting out. If you are ever constipated, this is the thing to do. About an hour after the internal saltwater bath, you have your first bowel movement. This is the first of many times in your ten-day cleanse that you will be surprised at how much is in your system. The saltwater really cleans you out and gets things moving. I chose to do the internal saltwater bath every morning rather than taking an herbal laxative; it just felt more natural to me.

After I did my internal saltwater bath and had my bowel movement, I was able to make my first official drink. I discovered that with each lemon I could get two 8-ounce drinks. I added all of the ingredients and took my first sip: Surprise! It actually tasted pretty good. I think having ripe lemons really helps.

I drank a total of eight lemonades the first day. I had several BMs, each very firm and dark in color. At the end of the first day, I was hungry but not starving. We took our son trick-or-treating—I was eager for the day to end so that all candy could be put away.

Day Two

I woke up, mixed the saltwater and drank it. It is not easy trying to drink the saltwater in a short amount of time, but I still prefer it over the herbal laxatives. About an hour later, I had my morning bowel movement. It was very dark in color and smelled downright toxic; I found myself debating purchasing a gas mask for the next nine days. My BMs so far were dark and very strong in smell.

After the saltwater bath, I drank the first of many lemonades for the day. I find that eight glasses a day keeps me going. I was still not dying from hunger as I thought I would be. I was feeling light-headed, and I had a slight headache the whole day. I found that I was able to continue with my daily routine minus the exercising. I was not one of the ones who had tons of energy on this cleanse; I kept everything at a bare minimum.

Day Three

Same routine with the internal saltwater bath first thing in the morning. Today I noticed that my BMs were starting to become looser and lighter in color. There seemed to be mucus, which freaked me out just a little. I picked up my book to make sure that I had read correctly and this was actually supposed to be happening. When I was done reading, I felt confident I was doing the right thing.

I still had a slight headache and felt light-headed. I seemed to be having trouble focusing. There was a part of me that wanted to eat something, but I knew if I did I would ruin what I had started. I of course chose not to eat anything, and I resisted taking anything to help with my headache.

I became very curious as to what toxins my body was trying to eliminate. I started to notice a foul smell coming from my body. I went to my husband and asked him to smell me. He took a whiff and confirmed that, yes, I did stink. The smell was not a typical body odor; it reminded me of what an elderly person smells like when they are on all types of medication. It was odd to me that the smell reminded me of medication because I am not on a regular medication. Had my body been holding on to medication that I had taken over the years? Frightening.

On this day I also learned the lesson to never leave home without a prepared drink. It's safe to say that I almost chewed my own arm off because I left home unprepared. After this experience, every time I left the house I prepared a drink and brought it with me in a stainless-steel container. (I used the special container because I was worried about the enzymes breaking down if they were exposed to the sun.) I also avoided leaving home for extended periods of time.

Day Four

As usual, I did my internal saltwater bath in the morning. I had my BM, and there was more mucus like yesterday. I was also starting to have a vaginal discharge throughout the day. I still had a slight headache and felt light-headed. I took my son for his playdates and continued my life as normal. Four days into the cleanse, I was a hundred percent committed to finishing; I knew that I could do this. I even made up a chart to display on the refrigerator for the ten-day countdown. I involved my son and asked him to put an "X" in a box every morning to show that Mommy had completed another day. He enjoyed this because it's what we do with him when he has a goal to attain. To him, my chart was as important as his potty-training chart.

On the chart, I started to keep track of the number of drinks I consumed each day and how many BMs I had. Believe me, this stuff becomes very important when you are doing the cleanse. If you've ever had an issue with looking in the toilet, you are going to have to throw that out the window. As you get further into the cleanse, you are going to be stunned at what actually comes out of your body.

Day Five

Again I did my morning internal saltwater bath and had my first BM of the day. I was starting to have more vaginal discharge. It was clear and goopy, not your normal discharge; I had to start wearing panty-liners because of the sheer volume. I found myself getting a little concerned about this, but my husband reassured me that my body would not get rid of anything I needed. I was unable to find much information in my book to explain the discharge. The book mentions mucus coming out of your sinuses and throat. I've never had any issues with my sinuses or throat; however, I have been "cursed" with female reproductive problems, including issues with my menstrual cycle, my whole life. I started to wonder if this mucus/discharge had something to do with the problems I'd had for all these years.

Around lunchtime, I decided to take my son on a shopping trip to Costco. If you're a mom, you know that Costco is a great place to feed your child with samples and then hope that they fall asleep on the way home. Well, on this particular shopping trip, I discovered the evils of Costco samples! Around every turn there was a table with delicious-smelling samples. I didn't even lick my fingers after giving my son his samples, in case I would be tempted. I purchased what I needed and made this my shortest Costco trip ever.

Day Six

I woke up feeling pretty good. I noticed that my skin was incredibly clear and my eyes were the most vibrant blue they had ever been.

Today was the day I realized what a test the Master Cleanse can be. On this day, my bowel movements really started to change. They became even lighter in color, and I saw that there was something in the toilet that resembled a molted snake skin or a sausage skin. It was about eight inches long, in what seemed to be the shape of a small intestine. I tried to tell myself that this was a "cast" of the lining of my intestine, but I couldn't help wondering if it was part of a parasite. To my surprise, I was fascinated. I wanted to call my husband at work and tell him, but then I thought maybe he wouldn't appreciate it as much as I did. It sounds crazy, but you actually find yourself wanting to share your most private experiences with everyone when you're on this cleanse. (You'll also want to persuade everyone important in your life to do the Master Cleanse for themselves.)

Throughout the day I continued to have BMs with what appeared to be sausage skin or a parasite. I was also still having the vaginal discharge. It had gotten heavy again and I was having to wear a panty-liner.

Day Seven

I woke up and went through my morning routine. By this time my son had grown completely accustomed to what was taking place in our home, and he was patient with my morning routine. I allowed him to help prepare my drinks so he could feel he was a part of what I was doing. I feel strongly that your children will grow up to care for themselves as you have modeled for them. I explained to him that Mommy was trying to make her body strong for another baby. This really spoke volumes to him because he is always asking for a sibling. I wondered to myself, what if I am giving this poor child false hope and we are unable to conceive another baby? What if I am giving myself false hope? I have learned that as a parent you are always second-guessing yourself.

During the seventh day I was still having the same type of BMs as the day before. They still looked like sausage skin. I was also having a lot of vaginal discharge/mucus. I continued with my daily routine. I found that taking a nap during dinner really helped with my hunger. My husband had told me that I was getting a little cranky and difficult to live with, so he was very happy with my decision to take a nap while he prepared dinner.

Day Eight

On the eighth day I had a regularly scheduled appointment with my general practitioner. When the nurse weighed me, he noticed I had lost ten pounds since the month before, when I was there for my knee. The nurse then took my blood pressure, which he found was too low.

I wasn't worried about that because my blood pressure is always very low; it runs in my family. When my doctor finally made it into the room, she too noticed my weight loss and became concerned. I assured her that I was fine, and I told her about the Master Cleanse. She started to scold me, telling me that I needed to stop the cleanse immediately and that she couldn't encourage any diet that does not involve food. I explained to her that I was getting my calories from the maple syrup, but she was not satisfied with my argument. As I left the appointment I felt a little deflated. I do respect my doctor's advice, but I also knew that what was happening with my body was a good thing.

After the doctor's appointment, I went to my MOPS (Mothers of Preschoolers) meeting. There are about sixty of us in this group. We meet twice a month and we know each other very well. When I walked in, the girls started remarking on how great I looked and how vibrant my eyes were. They all wanted to know what treatment I was using on my skin because it looked flawless. I told them about the cleanse and described what had just taken place at my doctor's appointment. The girls said they thought I would be crazy to stop the cleanse. It felt great to have my girl-friends encourage me and even say they wanted to do the cleanse themselves. (I held back on the gory details about the vaginal discharge and the BMs. I felt it would be better to discuss that within a smaller group, and I figured if they read the book they would learn that for themselves!) By the time I left the meeting I was no longer feeling deflated but, rather, determined.

Day Nine

I would be lying if I told you I wasn't ready for some food on Day Nine.

On this day, the vaginal discharge was becoming much lighter in volume. My BMs were light in color and there seemed to be no more lining of the intestines or parasites. I was feeling good. I can definitely see why you have to do this for at least ten days. If I had quit in the middle it would have been a shock to my system, bringing all of the toxins to the surface and then not allowing them to be expelled.

Day Ten

Tenth and final day—I did it! I was so happy and proud of myself. I lost a total of twelve pounds, my eyes were super-vibrant blue, and my skin looked better than it had ever looked since I was five. I did my normal routine with the saltwater and had my usual number of drinks for the day. My BMs were clear and the same as yesterday; I had no vaginal discharge.

My son was excited that today Mommy could fill her chart with X's. He wanted to know which toy Mommy would get to pick out at the toy store. It touched me that he was proud of me and wanted me to have a reward.

After the Cleanse

After my final day of the cleanse I was feeling excited about having food. I started with a mushroom-broth soup for the first day. It is suggested that you only drink orange juice, but this was too strong for me; it gave me a bit of an upset stomach.

To my surprise, I was not craving my typical diet, which includes carbohydrates and some processed foods. My body was screaming for raw foods. In my first few days off the cleanse, I started making an organic veggie soup that I still crave five months later. I have found that now when I eat processed foods I feel sluggish, almost as if my body wants to get rid of them ASAP. I have stopped eating most processed foods and I feel much better.

Since my cleanse, a lot has happened for our family. I started the cleanse October 31 and five weeks later we found out I was pregnant! I couldn't believe it. I must have conceived immediately after the cleanse. I know that it happened right after the cleanse because I was insistent on not having intercourse during the cleanse, thinking that it could possibly be another thing my body would have to try and eliminate.

A few weeks later, I had another appointment with my general practitioner about my knee. I told my doctor I was pregnant and went into detail about what had taken place during my cleanse. I told her about all the vaginal discharge/mucus that had come out of my body and how I thought this was related to my difficulty getting pregnant. To my great surprise, she congratulated me and actually agreed with me. She said that the mucus had most likely been coating my cervix and preventing me from getting pregnant. She then went on to explain that as a doctor of Western medicine she has been trained to discourage any type of alternative medicine or health practices. She gave me a huge hug and said, "Good job!"

Sadly, I miscarried ten weeks into the pregnancy. When we went to our routine appointment with the obstetrician, we found out that the fetus did not have a heartbeat. It was devastating. I did not have any bleeding at this time, and I chose to let the baby pass naturally instead of doing the recommended D&C. I had read that a D&C can create scar tissue and make it difficult to get pregnant again. When the baby still had not passed five days later, on Christmas Eve, I went to a dear friend who is an acupuncturist and asked him to perform acupuncture on me to help facilitate the miscarriage. He was able to do a specific point prescription that is frequently used in Chinese medicine for these situations. I felt nauseous as I was leaving his house, and this lasted throughout the evening. I also had a slight backache and general discomfort. Six hours after the acupuncture, I passed the fetus. I grieved for our loss; however, I still felt very hopeful. I kept thinking that if I was able to get pregnant immediately after the cleanse, maybe it could happen again. I even considered doing another cleanse, but I just didn't have it in me. I felt emotionally drained from the miscarriage.

Life continued, and eight weeks later we found out we were pregnant again! I had thought I was suffering from a bad case of the flu for a couple of weeks but my husband suggested we do a pregnancy test. I thought he was crazy and I didn't have the emotional strength to have the test come up negative. I finally agreed to do a home pregnancy test, but I asked my husband to be the one to look at the results. Well, it was positive. We were both stunned. How could this be, right after a miscarriage? When I went for an appointment with my obstetrician, I was amazed to find out that I was seven weeks pregnant.

We were very cautious with this pregnancy and chose not to tell our son or many friends, just in case something were to go wrong. Well, we are now into our second trimester and everything looks great! I would like to mention that my food cravings with this pregnancy are much different than with my son's pregnancy. During my first pregnancy I craved heavy foods, like homemade macaroni and cheese, doughnuts and Mexican food. Now I only want fresh veggies and fruit. I have to remind myself daily to eat enough calories to support the baby!

As you can see, I have had great success because of the cleanse. I would encourage any woman having difficulty getting pregnant to try this cleanse. It may not work for you, but it is only ten days—and if it does work, it could very easily change your life forever.

PART 3

Your Journal

As you prepare to embark on your own Master Cleanse, consider keeping a Master Cleanse journal. The final pages have been set aside for you to record your experiences, triumphs, strategies and trials of getting through this ten-day diet. After all, your Master Cleanse experience may just revolutionize your entire being, and that's something to remember.

Day One:

_____

_____

_____

_____

_____

_____

_____

_____

_____

_____

_____

_____

_____

_____

_____

_____

_____

_____

Your Journal

Day Two:

_____

_____

_____

_____

_____

_____

_____

_____

_____

_____

_____

_____

_____

_____

_____

_____

_____

_____

_____

Your Journal

Day Three:

_____

_____

_____

_____

_____

_____

_____

_____

_____

_____

_____

_____

_____

_____

_____

_____

_____

_____

Your Journal

Day Four:

_____

_____

_____

_____

_____

_____

_____

_____

_____

_____

_____

_____

_____

_____

_____

_____

_____

Day Five:

_____

_____

_____

_____

_____

_____

_____

_____

_____

_____

_____

_____

_____

_____

_____

_____

_____

Day Six:

_____

_____

_____

_____

_____

_____

_____

_____

_____

_____

_____

_____

_____

_____

_____

_____

_____

_____

Your Journal

Day Seven:

_____

_____

_____

_____

_____

_____

_____

_____

_____

_____

_____

_____

_____

_____

_____

_____

_____

Day Eight:

_____

_____

_____

_____

_____

_____

_____

_____

_____

_____

_____

_____

_____

_____

_____

_____

_____

_____

_____

_____

_____

_____

Your Journal

Day Nine:

Your Journal

Day Ten:

_____

_____

_____

_____

_____

_____

_____

_____

_____

_____

_____

_____

_____

_____

_____

Your Journal